The Didactics of Acute Lung Inflammation

The Didactics of Acute Lung Inflammation

By

Igor Klepikov

Cambridge Scholars Publishing

The Didactics of Acute Lung Inflammation

By Igor Klepikov

This book first published 2022

Cambridge Scholars Publishing

Lady Stephenson Library, Newcastle upon Tyne, NE6 2PA, UK

British Library Cataloguing in Publication Data
A catalogue record for this book is available from the British Library

ISBN (10): 1-5275-8810-6
ISBN (13): 978-1-5275-8810-3

This book is dedicated to my beloved daughters Yulia and Elena, who are always a source of inspiration in my work.

TABLE OF CONTENTS

Abbreviations

AP-acute pneumonia;

ARDS - Acute respiratory distress syndrome;

BSC - body surface cooling;

CAP-community-acquired pneumonia;

COVID-19 – coronavirus disease;

CPT – cupping therapy;

CRPG – comparative reopulmonography;

CVSB- cervical vagosympathetic blockade;

EP - Empyema of the pleura;

GBC - general body cooling;

HR - heart rate;

ICU- intensive care unit;

K v/p - coefficient of ventilation-perfusion ratio;

LG - lung gangrene

MBF - minute pulsatory blood flow;

MERS - Middle East respiratory syndrome;

MRSA - methicillin-resistant Staphylococcus aureus;

MTS – microtracheostomy;

MV - minute volume of ventilation;

PE - pulmonary embolism;

PM – Pneumomediastinum;

PP – Pneumopericardium;

RPG – reopulmonography;

RR – respiratory rate;

RV - respiratory volume;

SA - systolic wave amplitude;

SARS - severe acute respiratory syndrome;

VATS - video-assisted thoracic surgery

From the Author

The successes and achievements of modern medicine surprisingly bypass the actual and widespread problem of acute inflammatory processes of lung tissue. In this section of medicine, the situation has not only not changed for many years, but, according to statistics, it tends to gradually and steadily worsen. This is all the more strange because acute pneumonia is considered one of the oldest nosological forms, which has been observed and studied throughout the entire historical period.

In medicine, there is a wise and business tradition to bring all controversial and unresolved problems to public discussion, as well as to present the results of their own research to a wide audience. The information below is a combination of these circumstances. Unlike the vast majority of works published on this topic and devoted to its currently relevant features and details, in this case we are talking about the principles of solving the problem, which depend on the existing concept of the disease. It is the strategy of solving the problem that determines the direction of scientific research and the success of applying the results obtained. Mistakes and misconceptions that arise in the process of forming general ideas about the subject of attention are the main obstacle to achieving the goal.

Attention is drawn to the origins of those didactic distortions that formed the problem of acute inflammation of the lung tissue in its current form. No matter how unexpected and stunning it may sound, but the main reason for the current state of this problem is connected with one of the greatest discoveries of medicine of the last century, which are antibiotics. The phenomenal success of this antimicrobial therapy has narrowed the idea of the essence of the disease to the leading role of its causative agent. Today, this interpretation of the causes of pneumonia, despite significant changes in its etiology, remains an anchor that does not allow to move this problem from its place, and antibiotics, having lost their broad significance and initial effectiveness, continue to figure in the image of the main hope.

The modern ideology of acute inflammation of the lung tissue has been formed for many years under the influence of the priority of antibiotics. At present, firmly internalized stereotypes continue to serve as the basis for finding solutions in new situations and are not questioned, despite the presence of inconsistencies and refuting facts.

This feature of the problem under discussion goes beyond the scope of clinical medicine and is already an object of study in other disciplines. Such misconceptions, which gradually cover the consciousness and perception of an increasing part of society, despite the contradiction with existing facts and circumstances, are defined in modern psychology and sociology as a *"destructive meme"*. The ability of such defective material to further spread is designated by the term *"information cascade"*. These are just the factors that can serve as a vivid example of the psychological consequences of the use of antibiotics. However, the purpose of this work relates exclusively to the affected clinical topic, especially since the author is not a professional psychologist.

The information presented below includes, first of all, fundamental, well-known materials of medical science, which underlie professional ideas about inflammation and dysfunction of the affected organ, but which are not given sufficient attention in the modern concept of the disease. These materials were supplemented with the results of special studies and clinical trials.

Taking into account the imperative of the generally accepted concept of the disease in modern healthcare systems, as well as the fact that the duties of doctors and the limits of medical actions in any region of the world are determined by local laws and regulations, this manuscript is offered as an informational message. Such material for reflection is necessary today and will be useful to every specialist related to the section of acute inflammatory processes of the respiratory system. The proposed information summarizes the facts and objective evidence of existing inconsistencies and contradictions in understanding the nature of acute pneumonia, which during the SARS-CoV-2 pandemic turned into a diagnosis that frightens patients and causes pessimism among medical personnel.

Today, emergency care for patients with severe pneumonia is based on analogies with other inflammatory diseases, including terminology and causes of common complications. Monitoring of the condition of patients and evaluation of the effectiveness of treatment in patients with acute pulmonary pathology is carried out according to the same standards as in other variants of inflammatory processes. A common way to determine the effect of the tested therapy is to compare the dynamics of various cellular and molecular constants in the body, which do not allow us to assess the impact of a particular technique on the dynamics of the process and do not always reflect its clinical effectiveness.

Emergency care methods, which are currently widespread in patients with acute pneumonia, are palliative and supportive treatment. Modern treatment of such patients, especially with aggressive development of the disease, does not guarantee a favorable outcome, and often the negative dynamics of the process is observed against the background of intensive treatment and despite it. One of the main axioms of medicine, reflecting its purpose throughout history, says: if treatment does not bring relief to the patient and even more so does not prevent the further development of the disease, then such assistance does not correspond to the nature of the process, does it? This is one of the main issues underlying the following text.

In the current situation, the proposed information should serve as a reason to change the principles of monitoring patients with acute pneumonia. In particular, it is necessary to shift the priorities of control towards the dynamics of the main process and especially blood flow in the small circle of blood circulation, and not on the periphery, as it is customary to assess now, fixing attention on the consequences of the process instead of its main mechanisms. Such monitoring will first of all help to understand the reasons why the results of modern treatment of this category of patients do not have the desired effectiveness.

The general consequences of prolonged use of antibiotics are a topic of separate discussion, but the impact of this type of therapy on the problem of acute inflammation of the lung tissue, including its terminology, turned out to be more noticeable and tangible than in other diseases. Various variants of the designation of one process, such as community-acquired pneumonia, hospital pneumonia, COVID-19 pneumonia and others, are the product of the microbiological theory of the disease that dominates today and reflect mainly the supposed etiological characteristics, and not the scientific essence of the problem. Therefore, the following materials are purposefully devoted to one nosological form of the disease, which has been known to medicine throughout its centuries-old history as *"acute pneumonia"* (AP).

The term "AP" is used in the text as a single reflection of this nosological form, which continues to be divided into various variants in accordance with the assumed etiology. Modern classifications are declarative in nature and do not bring real practical benefits, pursuing only the choice of etiotropic therapy and concentrating all attention on one of the fragments of the whole problem. The absence of accurate and reliable differences in AP depending on the etiology of the process indicates the general basis of the disease, regardless of the pathogen. Various terms in the text are used only to denote information that is discussed in a particular fragment, and repeated descriptions of some materials allow us to show in more detail their significance in the overall process and their relationship with other factors.

The work, the results of which formed the basis of the information presented below, was started more than 40 years ago, so its results may cause distrust and doubts about their significance and reliability for modern conditions. At that time, the author found himself in a situation where the local geography of aggressive forms of AP and the concentration of such patients in one department was an unusual and unique phenomenon. Over the past decades, there have been changes in the development of this disease, which have led to the spread of similar situations around the world.

The role of viruses in the development of AP has increased significantly. The inability to clearly separate the bacterial and viral forms of the disease led during the SARS-CoV-2 pandemic to the need for widespread use of antibiotics and concentration of patients with AP in specialized departments. The phenomenon of combining severe patients in one workspace made it possible to more clearly see the insufficient effectiveness of medical care, but the general principles of solving this problem and the desire to find a way out of the current situation remained the same as forty years ago.

The purpose of the information presented below is to draw the attention of a wide range of specialists to distortions of the essence of the AP problem, which contradict the basic medical and biological laws and real facts. Among the various factors of the development and course of the disease, a clear preference is given to the pathogen, and the probability of success is inextricably linked with the hopes for etiotropic therapy. The persistent desire to succeed with the help of learned patterns and schemes that have developed over the period of antibiotic use, in fact, leave unclaimed the unique features of the pathogenesis of the disease.

Over the past decades, one can observe a periodic change of the leading pathogens of AP, the appearance of which adds a new terminology to the classification of the disease, reflecting its etiology, but does not change the foundations of this nosology. So, recently the term "COVID-19 pneumonia" has become widespread, which does not have clear differential diagnostic differences from bacterial forms of the disease (with the exception of microbiological tests). The mechanisms of the pathological process that distinguished AP from other localizations of inflammation have been the main characteristic of this disease throughout its history and will influence the features of its course regardless of our perception. The preservation of the current concept of AP only complicates the situation and makes it difficult to find a rational solution to this problem.

INTRODUCTION

WHY IS SUCH A BOOK NEEDED?

Among the nosologies known to modern medicine, acute pneumonia (AP) is one of the most ancient. Throughout its long history, AP has been considered a formidable disease with a severe course and high mortality. The unprecedented successes of the last few decades in many areas of medicine, the achievement of a fantastic level of modern diagnostics and pharmacology, impressive progress in the technical support of all stages of medical care create today, especially among residents of developed countries, an aura of reliability of health systems and a sense of confidence in the effective elimination of most existing threats to our health. This belief is not only fully justified, but also has read confirmation by the results of prevention and treatment of various pathologies.

But, it is only necessary to switch attention to the topic of AP, and you can see a situation that today does not correspond to positive assessments in any way. For many recent years, the results of AP treatment reflect a decrease in the effectiveness of medical care with a gradual increase in the number of complications and an increase in mortality rates. A more detailed analysis of the state of this problem shows that various attempts that have been made in recent decades to change this negative trend have failed to slow down this course. The current situation in this section of medicine creates a very real impression that the long history of acquaintance with this disease has not helped much in its study, and the rise of medical science and its successes bypass the affected topic.

Currently, AP remains one of the leading problems of medicine in all regions of the world, including developed countries with the most advanced healthcare systems and the latest achievements of medical science. The effectiveness of modern AP treatment is most accurately characterized by mortality rates that reflect situations lost by medicine. Thus, according to the World Health Organization, in 2016, 3 million people worldwide died from lower respiratory tract infections, the main place among which is occupied by AP (1). Among other diseases included in the infectious group, AP ranks first in the number of deaths, which account for 5% for outpatient patients, 12% for hospitalized patients and reach 30% for those who are placed in intensive care units (2).

It should be noted that for many decades, antibiotics were considered the main treatment for AP, but their effectiveness gradually decreased. In this regard, many efforts have been made in recent years to identify the microbe responsible for the disease, in order to start targeted treatment as early as possible. For this purpose, acute inflammatory processes in the lungs began to be divided into separate subgroups in accordance with the conditions in which the disease develops, which implies the probability of different etiologies of AP. Therefore, one of the most "mild" types of AP is the so-called community-acquired pneumonia (CAP), the mortality rates from which have just been presented above. Other variants of AP provided for by this classification, such as, for example, hospital-acquired or ventilator-associated pneumonia, occur, as can be seen from the names, in more difficult conditions and have an even higher mortality rate.

The fact that acute inflammation of the lung tissue remains in the group of the main causes of death for an infinitely long time is the basis for a deep and comprehensive analysis in order to clarify the factors of such stability. For example, in the United States of America, AP is constantly among the ten most deadly nosologies (3), and in Europe it is the fifth most important cause of death (4). These indicators demonstrate the situation in the most prosperous regions of the planet. If we make such calculations on the scale of the world community, then, as the WHO materials show, acute lower respiratory tract infections occupy the fourth place among the causes of death of people (5).

The above statistics relate only to bacterial forms of AP, which, according to popular beliefs and general confidence, at this stage is provided with the highest possible level of medical care. At the same time, no one focuses on such a rather strange circumstance as the treatment of completely incomparable (except etiology) inflammatory diseases with one antibiotic. These drugs are considered as the main therapeutic agent for a wide range of processes, including AP, although they are used empirically, that is, mainly taking into account existing assumptions about the etiology of a particular case, experience, capabilities and preferences of the attending physician (6-10).

In addition to the peculiarities of the choice of antibiotics for patients with AP, it should be recalled that for many years the steady growth of viral lung infections has caused concern among specialists, and the number of cases of viral pneumonia reported annually has reached 200 million (11-13). This figure, which at the time of its publication accounted for almost half of all AP observations in the world, is twice (!) the annual number of people infected (!) during the current SARS-CoV-2 pandemic. At the same time, medicine is already familiar with the coronavirus and its consequences, which have caused at least two major epidemics - SARS and MERS (14). However, the observed trend of shifts in the etiology of AP did not entail a radical analysis, a change in the strategy of the disease and the resulting principles of treatment.

Despite the growing trend of viral etiology of AP, the focus continued to be on the bacterial factor, which remained the main goal of therapeutic efforts, and antibiotics continued to be considered the "cornerstone" of therapy for these patients (6,15). The appearance in such an atmosphere of a large number of patients with COVID-19 pneumonia, against the causative agent of which the main "anti-pneumonic" remedy turned out to be incapacitated, turned out to be unexpected for most specialists. The new conditions violated the previous treatment stereotypes, which were actually focused on the antimicrobial approach, and clearly demonstrated the lack of comprehensive treatment for this localization of inflammation.

The feeling of a sudden loss of rational treatment of AP today is the reason for the intensive search for new means of etiotropic effects, which continues to focus steadily on the leading role of the etiology of the disease and is carried out in a "combat situation". At the same time, as A. H. Attaway and co-authors rightly point out (16), modern respiratory care revolves around auxiliary measures.

Despite the dramatic transformation that occurred both with the etiology of the inflammatory process in the lungs and with its treatment, there were no significant changes in the statistical results during the SARS-CoV-2 pandemic. 80% of patients infected with coronavirus tolerate this contact on an outpatient basis and without special medical care. At the same time, at least a quarter of them learn about this event only through diagnostic tests, since they have no signs of the disease (17-20). It is easy to see that this is the same 80% as in the outpatient group among patients with CAP (2). The only difference is that during a pandemic, the total figure takes into account the number of infected people, while the CAP statistics show only cases of the disease.

The statistical proportions have hardly changed among hospitalized patients, who during the pandemic make up the same 20% of the total contingent of coronavirus infected as hospitalizations among patients with CAP. However, it is the results of inpatient treatment that are of greater interest for reflection, since it is possible to compare a group of patients with CAP who receive optimal treatment in accordance with modern standards, and patients with COVID-19 pneumonia, whose medical care is supportive and symptomatic. No matter how surprising the result of such a comparison may seem, the fact is obvious - there is no significant difference in the main statistical indicators. For example, the percentage of patients who need to be transferred to intensive care units and the mortality rate reaching 30-50% in both groups (21-29) require an in-depth analysis of the current situation.

Despite maintaining the stability of the main statistical indicators, the emergence of the SARS-CoV-2 pandemic has significantly worsened the psychological situation. If earlier the CAP refers to infectious diseases, but did not require strict epidemiological measures, now the rapid and easy spread of the coronavirus has forced them to comply. To the contagiousness of this infection was added the uncertainty of a favorable outcome in the case of the disease. Although we are talking only about the spread of the pathogen, and not about the transmission of inflammation of the lung tissue, but the usual hope for antibiotics has lost its relevance. Finally, the epidemiological situation forced to change the rules for hospitalization of patients with COVID-19 pneumonia. Now, severe respiratory patients began to concentrate in specialized departments for this pathology.

The organization of specialized departments to combat coronavirus was not just a heavy, but an extremely heavy burden for the medical staff working in them. If earlier such patients were distributed to different departments, which significantly reduced the atmosphere of tension, now there are clusters of the most severe clinical situations when each patient requires extreme attention and super-maximum efforts. The aggressive dynamics of the disease and the rapid change of situations in each patient require immediate solutions and timely correction, but, most importantly, the percentage of observations in which the efforts expended were unsuccessful turned out to be too high. A reflection of such organizational movements turned out to be a whole series of articles devoted to mental shocks and depressive moods among employees of such specialized units (30-36).

The author of these lines found himself in a similar situation at the dawn of his career. At that time, the world was gripped by the so-called "staphylococcal catastrophe". A large number of patients with severe forms of AP appeared, which more often affected children, were characterized by rapid development and high mortality, and pathogenic strains of staphylococcus were considered the cause of this. The provision of medical care to this contingent of patients in a large Siberian city, where the author began working, was put in critical conditions. Most of the small city hospitals where such patients were admitted were not ready to provide intensive care, which newcomers often needed. In this regard, the city health department decided to hospitalize all patients with aggressive onset of AP in the surgical department of a multidisciplinary hospital, which worked in close contact with the intensive care unit.

The only difference between the circumstances in which the author found himself and the current concentration of patients with COVID-19 pneumonia was the absence of an epidemic situation. Otherwise, the intense atmosphere of work was ensured by the presence of 10-15, and sometimes more than 20 severe patients with AP at the same time in the department.

It should be noted that the very change in organizational measures to provide medical care to patients with AP did not significantly affect the results of treatment. The most severe category of these patients had the opportunity to be in the best observation conditions for that time and received optimal treatment in accordance with international standards. However, the dynamics of inflammatory processes was characterized by aggressive development, rapid addition of pleural complications and high mortality, which exceeded 10%. Such results forced us to look for ways to improve the effectiveness of therapeutic measures, and the first doubts about the adequacy of the therapy arose at the moment of realizing that staphylococcus is not the main cause of such a severe and complicated course of AP.

While all the information on this problem presented staphylococcus as the main cause of the crisis, and the professional literature was overflowing with reports about the exceptional virulence of this pathogen and options for its suppression, the real facts contradicted the validity of such a concept. Bacteriological studies of purulent contents from the inflammatory zone already at the early stages of the disease revealed other types of pathogens, and often such material for research turned out to be sterile.

To the doubts that arose about the leading role of etiotropic treatment in AP, uncertainty was added in the correct choice of a number of treatment methods, which from general therapeutic practice were transferred to the exceptional conditions of localization of the focus of inflammation in the small circle of blood circulation. In the end, a lot of research work was started, which was based on a radical revision of the entire concept of AP. The result of this work and clinical approbation of pathogenetic principles of treatment was a unique success of therapy with the possibility of guaranteed prevention of complications of the disease.

The combination of a number of circumstances did not allow timely translation and presentation of the results achieved to a wide range of specialists at the international level. However, over the past period of time, inconsistencies between existing ideas about the nature of AP and real facts, which are especially inherent in the most acute forms of the disease, have not only not become a thing of the past, but, on the contrary, have become more pronounced. In this regard, the importance of the results of the work done earlier to solve the problem of AP in its current state has only increased.

It should be noted that in recent decades there has been a periodic change of the leading pathogens in the etiology of AP, which was reflected only in tactical nuances. The information base of scientific data on the topic under discussion has also expanded significantly in recent years, but the strategy for solving the problem has not changed. Today, the desire to find a universal drug that can help with the development of AP, especially with its aggressive course, and bring, if not instantaneous, then a very rapid positive effect, continues to prevail. Such illusory hopes were formed and strengthened in the process of reducing the effectiveness of antibiotics, stimulating the search for equivalent replacements, and continue to determine the directions of ongoing research under the influence of the established AP concept.

Today, a broad but fruitless search for etiotropic antiviral drugs continues in the hope of repeating the success of the initial use of antibiotics and again achieving a revolutionary breakthrough in the treatment of AP (37). However, the absence of direct parallels when comparing antibacterial and antiviral methods of exposure remains beyond the scope of discussion. Currently, efforts are being made to find therapeutic options for blocking the penetration of viruses into the cell. That is, there are searches for ways to prevent the disease, and not medical care when it occurs.

When viral pneumonia has already been diagnosed, by this time the virus has not only "hidden" in the cells, but also contributed to the development of inflammatory changes in tissue structures. Those manifestations of the disease that we can see and evaluate in clinical conditions are the result of organ damage and disruption of its functions, but not a reflection of the characteristics of the pathogen. After all, bacterial forms of pneumonia have similar manifestations, and therefore, in most cases, it is extremely difficult or impossible to make a differential diagnosis between them according to etiological signs, isn't it? Therefore, drugs that can prevent the virus from entering the cells can, at best, prevent the further spread of the process, but cannot provide the necessary therapeutic effect of the disorders that have already occurred.

Dreams of creating a universal etiotropic treatment for pneumonia largely determine today's plans and directions in solving the problem of AP. No, no one claims the need to develop a so-called "pneumonia pill", which a priori cannot exist in nature, but the main efforts of research and clinical trials are aimed at finding remedies against the pathogens of AP. Stereotypes of ideas that have arisen as a result of prolonged use of antibiotics continue to dominate the interpretation of changes occurring in the etiology of AP.

The exclusively antimicrobial effect of antibiotics was initially used as an additional agent in the treatment of AP, which corresponded to its main pharmacological characteristic. However, in the future, contrary to logic and professional ideas, this type of therapy began to be interpreted as the only and main method of treating acute nonspecific inflammation (!), and the initial treatment of patients with AP was for a long time designated by the term "antibiotics alone".

The periodic change of the main pathogens of AP observed in recent decades has clearly shown that the type of pathogen does not determine the severity of the course and features of the development of the disease. For example, clinical manifestations of bacterial forms of AP did not allow to determine the type of pathogen in each specific case for a targeted choice of antibiotics. Antimicrobial action as the basis for the treatment of this group of patients posed the task of accurately diagnosing the etiology of the process, which researchers had unsuccessfully tried to solve for many years, although the answer lay on the surface: the stability of the disease clinic, regardless of the etiology, was due to a constant violation of lung function as a result of the development of the inflammatory process.

Microbiological factors in the development of AP can influence certain nuances of inflammatory tissue transformation and some clinical and laboratory shades of the process, but even with the help of special diagnostic methods, it is not always possible to identify and determine those features that depend on the etiology of the disease, which is nonspecific in nature. At the same time, the focus of inflammation by its occurrence inevitably affects the function of the affected organ, determining, depending on the localization, all the further originality of the clinic. That's why inflammation in the lung cannot be confused with inflammation of another localization, for example, with osteomyelitis, sore throat or hepatitis, right?

A detailed acquaintance with the modern strategy for solving the problem of AP allows us to note that it is focused on the etiology of the disease, but does not attach due importance to a number of important axioms of medical science. Having recently received a large influx of patients with COVID-19 pneumonia and having lost the possibility of using specific treatment methods in this group of patients, medicine finally drew attention to the need to revise strategic directions for solving the problem. During the SARS-CoV-2 pandemic, publications with proposals for revising general approaches to helping with inflammatory lung processes became more frequent.

When the solution of the problem by existing methods does not bring the expected results, the analysis and revision of the current strategy is absolutely the right and logical step from which to begin the search for new developments. However, the materials proposed today concerning changes in strategic solutions to the AP problem actually contain only individual tactical techniques, while maintaining the suppression of the pathogen of the process as the main goal (38-44). Thus, in addition to the indicated desire to change the basis of strategic approaches to solving this problem, no real changes in the strategy have yet been proposed.

The strategy for solving the AP problem depends entirely on our conceptual ideas about the nature of the disease. The introduction of any new proposals to the list of therapeutic measures, the interpretation of their expected effect and even the explanation of the results of their testing will be determined by our understanding of the essence of the development of the process. At the same time, the process that has arisen will develop according to its biological laws, regardless of how we imagine and understand it, right? Such a course of events in the absence of additional external influences remains a natural variant of the development of the disease, which has its own individual characteristics.

However, when there is a need to provide medical care to patients with AP, professional recommendations are inevitably determined by prevailing ideas about the nature of the disease and, consequently, the existing concept. In this case, the treatment is an intervention in the natural course of the process, and its results will depend on the nature and direction of therapeutic actions. As experience and facts show, therapeutic measures can have a certain impact on the dynamics of the disease, and such an impact can be both positive and negative.

Thus, a detailed study of the causes that currently do not allow finding an effective solution to the problem of acute inflammation of the lung tissue shows that the main obstacle is the nature of the mental perception of the nature of the disease at the professional level. Justification of the existing misconceptions in this section of medicine, facts and objective evidence of such a conclusion are presented in the proposed publication. Such information is necessary today for a wide range of specialists related to this category of patients, and therefore the publication of the proposed materials should play the role of an explanatory manual, which is extremely necessary for understanding the current situation.

CHAPTER 1

A BRIEF HISTORY OF TREATMENT OF ACUTE PNEUMONIA

1.1. Pre-antibiotic period

AP has been familiar to medicine since the time of Hippocrates for more than two and a half millennia (45). However, despite such a long history and wide progress of medical science, the problem of effective treatment of these patients not only remains unresolved, but, contrary to logic and expectations, its relevance and acuteness in recent decades continue to grow worldwide.

Historical experience in any discipline is invaluable for its future, as studying the results of previous practice allows you to use and develop previous successes and achievements at a new level, but at the same time avoid the mistakes of the past. Looking from these positions at the current state of the AP problem, it seems that this disease, which has one of the longest histories in medicine, does not have worthy results of centuries of experience.

Today we can say with confidence that the history of AP treatment is divided into two fundamentally different periods. Initially, for many centuries, medicine scrupulously accumulated experience and information about methods of treating this disease. This lengthy process was purely empirical. The constructiveness of such searches was very difficult, unproductive and often tragic. The lack of basic medical knowledge and scientific ideas about the laws of the biological world, dubious plans and the lack of technical support for ongoing tests and research were difficult obstacles. Nevertheless, over a long period of time, certain medical traditions and a set of means of providing assistance to this category of patients have gradually developed.

If we try to draw analogies between ancient and modern medicine, then the former simply will not be able to compete with modern healthcare systems in terms of its cognitive, technical and other capabilities. However, in one comparative aspect, ancient medicine has, from my point of view, clear advantages.

In the old days, medicine was not able to conduct research at the microscopic and molecular level, so observations and studies were carried out in areas that do not require special equipment. The patient as an object of observation for a long time was not only the main, but also the only figure in the diagnostic and therapeutic process, and the main purpose of observations and the basis for conclusions were changes in the condition and well-being of a sick person, as well as violations of vital functions of his body.

The modern patient still remains the main object of medical care, but today his condition is largely perceived through the prism of diagnostic procedures, as a virtual totality and interaction of various cells, molecules and microscopic substances. Such an assessment is often carried out from the position of a narrow professional specialization, when many phenomena and reactions that partially reflect the mechanism of the disease begin to take on the form of leading and decisive.

Ancient medicine still had no idea about the so-called non-respiratory functions of the lungs and did not have information that one of the leading functions of this organ is related to blood circulation and its regulation, and that violation of these parameters occurs first. For example, shortness of breath may occur in the presence of a small focus of inflammation in the lungs, when it is difficult to explain a critical decrease in the area of alveolar gas exchange. Looking ahead, it can be noted that one of the reasons for the increase in the frequency of respiratory excursions is associated with a violation of the proportions between ventilation and blood flow, and today there are objective confirmations of the positive effect of some ancient procedures in such situations.

At the time of the development of the focus of inflammation in the lung, a sudden violation of blood flow in the small circulatory circle, the pressure in which, under normal conditions, is several times lower than in the periphery, causes the body to reduce venous return, preventing the growth of pulmonary edema. It seems that ancient medicine understood the mechanism of such adaptation better than modern medicine. Lacking the means and capabilities for accurate and objective measurement and monitoring in patients with AP, the old medicine empirically found ways to help the patient's body to equalize emerging disorders in the most critical situations. Of course, it was a difficult trial and error experience, which in itself took more than one life.

For example, today such a method of helping patients with AP as bloodletting is no longer used in official medicine, but in the past it was used quite widely (46). The very principle of this procedure was to rapidly reduce the volume of circulating blood and reduce its return to the small circle of blood circulation. The extracted blood was irretrievably lost to the patient's body, and there were no strict rules for performing this procedure, which can be noted from the description of individual observations that have come down to our days.

The following story from the past is very revealing. According to the narrative about the death of the first president of the United States of America, George Washington, his death was not without the influence of bloodletting (47). Most likely, signs of a severe cold with fever, chest pain and difficulty breathing could be associated with AP, but the exact diagnosis was never established. Feeling the first signs of malaise, the patient made himself the first bloodletting, which did not bring relief. An urgently invited commission of doctors carried out several more bloodletting in a short time, removing a total of more than half of the patient's circulating blood. Of course, it was done with the best intentions, although nowadays even paramedics know that such a volume of blood loss is incompatible with life.

The description of external bloodletting can be found even in fiction. For example, a couple of centuries ago, the world-famous French writer Alexandre Dumas-father noted in his works that with pneumonia, a wound in a duel with a small loss of blood was accompanied, oddly enough, by relief for the wounded. The odiousness of this technique would not allow it to be in demand in medicine for this category of patients for a long time if it did not have a hidden pathophysiological meaning and did not bring relief to those in need.

Approximately the same principle of action was the use of leeches, the formulation of which did not imply strict accounting of extracted and irretrievably lost blood for the body (48). Currently, this method of treatment has also lost its former popularity.

Procedures such as cupping therapy (49) and short-term cooling of the patient's body (50,51) can have an effect similar to external bloodletting, but without loss of the patient's own blood. These methods also have a centuries-old history of use in acute inflammation of the lung tissue, but their effect is more gentle and is aimed at internal redistribution of blood with its partial deposition.

Currently, cupping therapy and body cooling continue to be widely used, but outside of therapeutic medicine. These procedures can be found among the list of services in various fitness clubs, sports and beauty centers and firms, and their advantages are mainly explained on the basis of impressions, assumptions and even ancient considerations. Today, such arguments are clearly not enough to convince us of the effectiveness of these procedures.

Currently, cupping therapy belongs to the category of alternative medicine and receives diametrically opposite assessments - from complete denial of its medicinal properties to laudatory reviews. It is enough to recall the photo of 23-time Olympic champion Michael Phelps with traces of medical cans on his body, which was printed by the world's leading press in 2016. The purpose of this publication was due only to the non-standard nature of such photo information, since the purpose of using cans in a healthy athlete remained undisclosed, and it is difficult to assume the grounds for such therapy. In this context, we should not talk about the fashion for this procedure, but about an objective assessment of its therapeutic effect and the expediency of its use in patients with AP.

It should also be noted that cryotherapy (51), which uses ultra-low temperatures, is a relatively recent invention, although its extreme effects are based on the ancient experience of general cooling. In the old days, ice baths were used for medical purposes for many painful conditions, including hyperthermia and acute inflammatory processes of the lungs. Currently, general hypothermia in medical institutions is mainly used to perform a number of operations and treat terminal conditions. However, this cooling option has a completely different purpose. Such hypothermia is prolonged and is aimed at achieving a steady decrease in body temperature for a certain period, which reduces the overall level of metabolic processes and increases the viability of tissues in conditions of impaired nutrition.

The principles of general cooling, which are based on the effect of short-term exposure to low temperatures on the surface of the patient's body, are currently not included in the arsenal of official medicine. Various variants of these techniques have gained particular popularity among athletes and in the so-called health groups today. Traditional medicine has not yet shown interest in the study and application of such methods of assistance.

The possibility of applying some procedures of ancient medicine should be based on an understanding of their influence on certain links of pathogenesis, as well as on objective criteria for evaluating the effect of each such manipulation. This approach will make it possible to establish the feasibility of using a specific technique and clarify the indications and contraindications for its use. The current situation, in which the experience of ancient medicine is not even subjected to attempts to test its therapeutic capabilities, looks completely illogical. This is all the more incomprehensible when the modern medical industry cannot offer any ways to adapt the body to severe and aggressive functional disorders in patients with AP.

The above-mentioned list of techniques that originated in ancient times and have survived to the present day can probably be supplemented and continued. However, in this presentation, procedures were mentioned that, according to the author, may be more relevant to the topic as first aid measures. Other methods of treatment that were used during this period (for example, the application of tourniquets on limbs) did not have such a target value for patients of this category and were not widely popular. Drug therapy has also had no noticeable success in this direction.

1.2. The era of antibiotics

The second period in the history of the AP is radically different from its centuries-old chronicle. The discovery of antibiotics and the beginning of the use of this therapy in the middle of the last century radically changed not only the principles of treatment of this disease, but also had a very strong influence on the formation of professional ideas about it. It is no coincidence that the last few decades are often called the era of antibiotics.

The first successes of antibiotic therapy began to create the impression that medicine received a universal and effective treatment. This feeling continued to grow despite the emergence of antibiotic-resistant strains, the decline in the effectiveness of drugs and the need for their constant updating. Antibiotics continued to save many patients, and in this atmosphere of momentary luck there was no place for a critical and balanced prognosis of the long-term consequences of such "sterilizing" therapy. The centuries-old experience of helping these patients was no longer taken into account, and his methods were discarded even without attempts to test their possible effect.

Antibiotics, despite their obvious side effects, have firmly taken the place of the main, and often the only means in the treatment of patients with AP. For a long time, the initial treatment of this category of patients was defined by the term "antibiotics alone". The short-sightedness of such a strategy became more and more obvious every year, but the desire to defeat the disease with the help of antibiotics only grew. The belief in the indispensability of this type of therapy has grown with each new generation of doctors.

Over time, the use of antibiotics and their effect on the microflora that accompanies our body has significantly expanded not only as a result of medical prescriptions. For example, many people know about the use of these drugs in such branches of the food industry as animal husbandry, poultry farming and even fishing. In this regard, many countries have adopted laws and regulations that oblige manufacturers to provide information about the use of these medicines in the production of the final product (Figure 1). The widespread and long-term use of antibiotics could not remain without biological consequences, which continue to progress slowly but steadily.

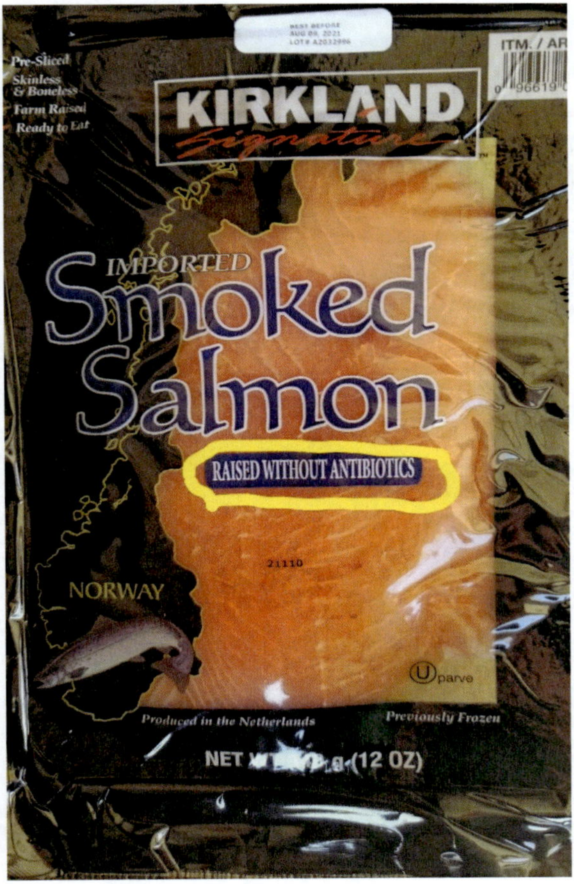

Figure 1. Food packaging with information about the use of antibiotics in the production process.

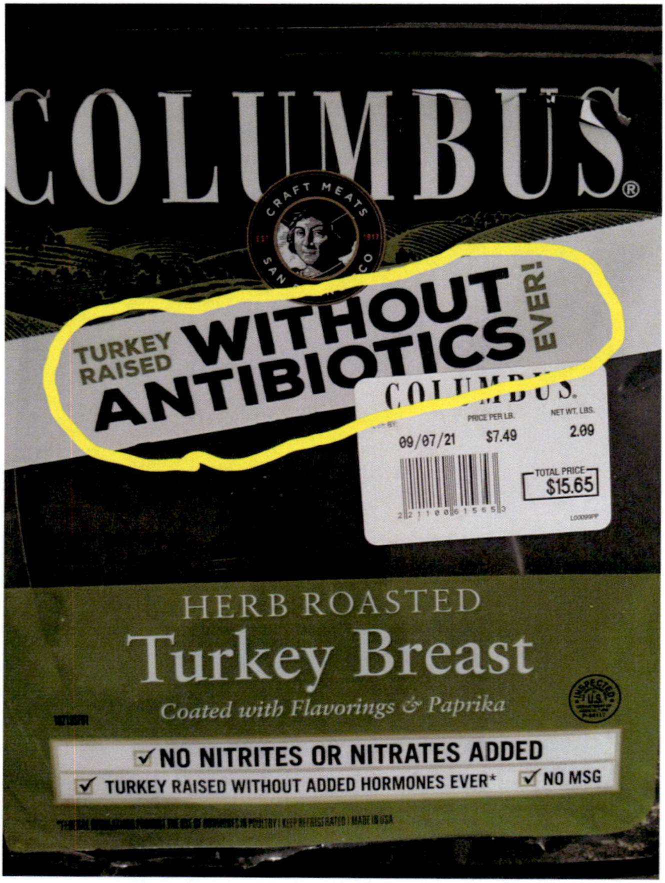

Figure 1 (continued). Food packaging with information about the use of antibiotics in the production process.

Antibiotics are still one of the most popular medications, and almost one in five prescriptions (19%) of these drugs are prescribed to patients with AP (52). Their action, unlike other representatives of the pharmacopoeia, is directed not at the structures and substances of the body, but at its microflora. It is this circumstance that can explain the paradox that the same antibiotic is able to help as a general therapeutic agent for diseases that are completely incomparable with each other. At the same time, each representative of the microbial world is in itself a separate biological object with such a quality as adaptability.

The latter circumstance makes it possible to understand the causes of the consequences of antibacterial therapy and the unreality of its infinite effectiveness. Moreover, the long-term and widespread, but not always controlled (as, for example, in the food industry) use of antibiotics not only changed the qualitative characteristics of individual strains, but also affected the habitual balance between the body and its accompanying microflora. In this regard, it is necessary to pay attention once again to the steady growth of viral inflammation of the lung tissue in recent decades (11-13). Annual severe flu epidemics have become commonplace. The "suddenness" of the current SARS-CoV-2 pandemic was preceded by two major coronavirus epidemics (SARS, MERS), the consequences of which did not affect the strategy and tactics of AP treatment.

The influence of antibiotics on the increasing role of viruses in the development of inflammatory processes of the lungs still remains a postulate. This fact is supported only by a noticeable decrease in the therapeutic effectiveness of antibiotics and a statistical trend in the growth of diseases of viral etiology. However, the latest data cannot be considered convincing proof of this opinion. On the other hand, there are no noticeable prerequisites for refuting this conclusion. To obtain weighty arguments, additional evidence is needed, such as, for example, an assessment of the dynamics of the microbiome of the human body and the percentage ratio between bacteria and viruses. In addition, when clarifying the essence of this postulate, time, as always, can play the role of an arbitrator in solving this dilemma.

In addition to the biological consequences of the use of antibiotics, they have had a very significant impact on professional views regarding the essence and nature of AP. Today, as in the initial period of the use of antibiotics, their positive effect is considered as the main condition for success in the treatment of AP. Even in situations where the source of inflammation is a virus and there are no signs of bacterial infection, antibiotics continue to be actively and widely used in treatment (6-10).

In this regard, it is again necessary to recall the purpose of antibacterial therapy, which is moving further away from the essence of such a disease as AP. This type of drugs can affect the bacterial factor of inflammation only if it is one of the causes of the disease and when the pathogen is sensitive to the selected drug. This is an axiom of this type of treatment. However, the basis of the disease, which consists of morphological and functional disorders as a result of the inflammation that has arisen, with such a narrow direction of help, completely depends on the elimination by the body itself.

In recent years, in the literature devoted to the problem of AP, such a term as "antibiotics alone" has already ceased to flash. The period when prescribing antimicrobial therapy was enough for many patients to achieve the desired result is in the past. The gradual decrease in the activity of this therapy every year more and more required the use of additional means of treatment. This applies, first of all, to patients in case of their hospitalization. However, by this time there was already a stereotype of ideas that bacteria play a leading role in the development and dynamics of AP. The significance and peculiarity of the mechanisms of the disease, which have fundamental differences from other inflammatory processes, remained out of sight, and therefore additional means of assistance began to be used by analogy with the general therapeutic experience of treatment.

In the end, a long period of antibiotic use led not only to the biological consequences of this method, but also to a serious distortion of ideas about the nature of AP. The concepts of the disease that exist today and the principles of medical care that follow from them do not agree with a number of classical materials of medical science. To understand what these misconceptions are and what role they play in the current state of the AP problem, a more detailed analysis is needed, which is presented in the next chapter.

CHAPTER 2

MODERN MYTHS ABOUT ACUTE PNEUMONIA

The order of presentation of the materials in this chapter does not reflect their significance for the problem under discussion, since the sections presented below are closely interrelated, being separate links of the general doctrine of the disease. They are presented approximately in the sequence that is accepted in the general description of the AP in textbooks and manuals.

2.1. Is AP an infectious disease?

Throughout the centuries-old history of the AP, there has been no evidence of the contagiousness of this disease and the danger of its transmission from a sick person to a healthy one. People who became ill with AP were not subjected to isolation and other precautions necessary for infectious processes. There was only a certain seasonal difference in the frequency of this disease, but no epidemics of AP were observed.

The development of microbiology, which arose much earlier than the appearance of antibiotics, did not affect the interpretation of AP, which continued to be considered as acute inflammation. With the discovery of *streptococcus pneumoniae* more than 140 years ago, it was found that it is the most frequent causative agent of AP, as a result of which it received the meaningful name "*pneumococcus*" (53). However, along with *pneumococcus*, inflammatory processes of the lungs could occur with the participation of other microorganisms, so for a long time the microbiological and pathological essence of the disease was precisely concentrated in the term "*acute nonspecific inflammation of the lungs*". In this name, the word "*nonspecific*" emphasizes the absence of a pathogen specific only to AP, as well as the fact that strains of microbes involved in inflammation of lung tissue can be found among symbionts in healthy people.

After the active use of antibiotics began, a new phenomenon appeared, which was not observed in the pre-antibiotic era. In this case, we are talking about a periodic and fairly obvious change of leaders among the agents of the AP. For example, if before the use of antibiotics, pneumococcus was the causative agent of AP in 90-95% of cases (403,471,472), then in recent years its participation in this disease has been confirmed only in 33-50% of positive bacteriological studies (473). However, if we calculate its presence among the total number of patients with AP, among whom in recent years it has not been possible to identify the pathogen in half or more cases, then the role of pneumococcus in the etiology of the disease is confirmed only in 10.9% of outpatient patients, in 17.7% of hospitalized and in 22.5% of these patients in intensive care units (474).

The place of pneumococcus, which began to disappear in the etiology of AP, began to be occupied by microorganisms that were found among the symbionts of the organism. Especially impressive was the surge of staphylococcal pneumonia, which peaked in the 60-70s of the last century. And yet the non-specificity and inconstancy of the etiology of AP contradict the fact that this inflammatory process, at least for the last two decades, has been regarded as an infectious disease. As an example, we can give a couple of brief quotations typical of scientific articles of recent years.

> *"Among infectious diseases, CAP is the most frequent cause of hospitalization and mortality in industrialized countries" (54).*

> *"Community-acquired pneumonia (CAP) is the infectious disease with the highest number of deaths worldwide" (55).*

This interpretation is all the more illogical because during this period there were no drastic changes in the epidemiology of AP. After staphylococcus unexpectedly became the sole leader among AP pathogens at first, and then lost this position, pneumococcus gradually returned to its usual place, although its advantage was significantly reduced, accounting for a third of observations among positive bacteriological tests (56-58). In addition, it should be added that in 62% of patients with AP, the pathogen remains unknown at all (2.59), and, according to some data, this indicator can range from 55 to 74% (60). How justified are the claims about the infectious nature of the disease, if information about the etiology remains unknown in most patients?

Epidemiological situation around patients with AP (before the coronavirus pandemic) it also did not change, and they were still in free mode. The only exceptions were patients who had an antibiotic-resistant flora. However, apart from the fact of this diagnosis and additional difficulties in choosing antimicrobials, no other special manifestations were observed in the treated patients. In addition, the probability of the presence of antibiotic-resistant strains among the symbiotic microflora in healthy people has already become a familiar fact, although such findings were not equivalent to a mandatory disease (61-63).

The distortion of views on the nature of AP occurred gradually along with a decrease in the effectiveness of antibiotics and an increase in the resistance of microflora. Acute inflammation of the lung tissue for a long time after the start of the use of antibiotics continued to be considered as a nonspecific inflammatory process, but not as an infectious disease. However, a further decrease in the effectiveness of antibiotics, instead of a critical reassessment of their place in the surrounding reality and the development of side effects, was accompanied by a growing desire to preserve their effectiveness. The tendency to solve the problem of AP with the help of etiotropic therapy has grown with each new generation of doctors, accustoming them to the idea of the leading role of the infectious principle in this disease.

The attribution of bacterial forms of AP to the category of infectious diseases is the result of a long and excessive perception of the role of antibiotics as the main means in the treatment process. The introduction of this term (infectious) in the description of the AP has no reasoned scientific basis and only further narrows the view of the problem, creating additional difficulties in solving it.

In this context, it is useful to recall the viral forms of AP, the pathogens of which have the ability to spread rapidly, which requires compliance with epidemiological measures. The frequency of viral lung lesions in recent decades has been characterized by an unprecedented increase in the entire history of AP (11-13), which not without reason allows us to consider this phenomenon as a natural consequence of prolonged exposure to antibacterial drugs. If earlier banal bacterial inflammations were often the result of respiratory viral diseases, during which the number of such patients increased, then in recent years the viral expansion has grown so much that the growth of these forms of AP in the autumn-winter period is already becoming an annual ritual, which periodically takes on the character of epidemics (14) and even pandemics.

With the viral etiology of AP, the term "infectious" may correspond to such characteristics of the disease as the ease of transmission of the pathogen and the need to comply with anti-epidemic measures. However, even the dangerous ease of infection does not mean a mandatory disease. According to the statistics of the current SARS-COV-2 pandemic, the causative agent of which experts assess as particularly virulent, the overwhelming number of infected people (up to 80%) overcome this contact without resorting to medical care, and in a fifth of them the infection usually remains asymptomatic (17-20).

Another block of accumulated information concerning AP is most directly related to the term "infectious". It is well known and proven by time that a revolutionary step in the prevention of many infectious diseases was made thanks to the development and implementation of vaccination. The modern interpretation of AP as an infectious disease suggested the idea of such vaccinations to prevent acute inflammation of the lung tissue. The rationale for such a company was based mainly on analogies and even assumptions.

In this regard, it is necessary to recall once again that true infectious diseases are distinguished by the strict specificity of their pathogen. The use of a specific vaccine in such situations guarantees almost absolute success. The cardinal distinguishing feature of AP is the absence of one specific pathogen. In the event of conditions for the development of AP, any of the potentially known pathogens can play the role of a trigger factor. To date, more than a hundred microorganisms involved in acute inflammatory processes in the lungs have been identified (64).

The latest information on the spectrum of etiological variants of AP should have raised the question of which specific pathogen a vaccine should be created against in order for its use to bring success. After all, AP didn't have such a separate pathogen before, and the list of the most active strains has been constantly changing lately. In this situation, the lot fell on the creation of an anti-pneumococcal vaccine. And although at the beginning of vaccination against pneumonia, according to available data, *streptococcus pneumoniae* prevailed among the pathogens, but initially such a campaign could not count on success similar to the prevention of other infections. The pneumococcal vaccine cannot cover most of the list of the most common pathogens of AP.

The first results of vaccination against pneumococcus raised a question that was not given a reasoned answer. Despite extensive and long-term vaccination, the number of patients with severe forms of AP did not decrease, and the number of pleural empyema among them increased statistically significantly (65,66). The analysis of the results of vaccination of the population against pneumonia according to the dynamics in the etiology of the disease is very indicative. For example, *pneumococci* and *haemophilus influenzae* decreased their presence among bacterial AP factors, but at the same time the participation of pathogens such as *Pseudomonas spp., Staphylococcus aureus* and *influenza virus* increased (67).

These materials indicate that pneumonia has its own menu of pathogens and the suppression of one of them, even the most active, does not affect the entire process of acute inflammation in the lungs. Such statistics, which often appear in the literature, are only additional evidence of groundless efforts to combat the selected pathogen of AP. One of the manifestations of the consequences of such a company was the so-called staphylococcal catastrophe, which was mentioned above and which arose after a decade of active use of antibiotics.

By choosing *Streptococcus pneumoniae* as the main target and using a specific vaccine against it for preventive purposes for more than 20 years, the medical scientific world has been convinced during this time that the effectiveness of the original version of this vaccine has significantly decreased. To increase its protective properties, a significant correction of this drug was required (68,69). Moreover, the proportion of *pneumococcus* in the etiology of AP has decreased significantly over the past period, and the latest versions of the vaccine require additional expansion of its range due to the appearance of new modifications of this microorganism (56-58). In other words, attempts to exterminate one of the bacterial pathogens of AP are accompanied by an increase in its resistance to external aggression factors and an increase in the role of other varieties from the list of microbiological causes of the disease.

The decrease in the overall incidence of AP, which was observed after the start of pneumococcal vaccination of the population, is not the result of a specific action of this procedure. Probably, this circumstance is due to some strengthening of the general nonspecific protection of the body, which, in conditions of a diverse and often unknown etiology, begins to bring at least a small effect. Nevertheless, pneumococcal vaccination does not guarantee the possibility of avoiding acute inflammation of the lung tissue, and in case of its development, the risk of severe complications has continued to grow in recent years. For example, in England and France, where vaccination of the population against pneumonia has been actively carried out for a long time, pleural empyema as a complication of AP continues to grow, and there are no reasoned explanations for this fact (70,71).

The presented point of view regarding "vaccination against pneumonia" finds unexpected and rather strong confirmation during the current SARS-CoV-2 pandemic. The presence of one causative agent of a new form of COVID-19 pneumonia gave hope in advance that the start of vaccination would radically change the dramatic development of this phenomenon. However, now that in many countries the majority of the population has been vaccinated, it has become quite obvious that vaccination reduces the risk of disease, but does not provide any guarantees of full protection. Moreover, to date, the list of newly ill and deceased among vaccinated people continues to be replenished, although their percentage, according to news reports, is lower than among unvaccinated citizens, but the analysis of generalizing statistics has not yet been given. Meanwhile, the lack of the expected effect of vaccination has caused booster injections, which have been started in many countries.

The above information confirms the old rule that says that people do not get infected with pneumonia, but get sick. Infection of the body means the transmission of a pathogen that does not belong to the representatives of our microbiota, but this fact is not equivalent to the transmission of the disease, since additional conditions are necessary for the development of AP. In this regard, the emphasis on the word "infection" has a double meaning. Such terminology is relatively important only for the epidemiology of viral diseases. At the same time, the general meaning of this term for all variants of AP plays only a negative role. Even without this terminology, AP pathogens are currently considered the only cause of the disease, which is incorrect. Therefore, additional emphasis on the etiology of the process will support and deepen this misconception.

2.2. Are the development and severity of AP due to the properties of its pathogen?

2.2.1. Formation of views on the etiology of AP

Information about AP pathogens began to accumulate with the advent and development of microbiology, and this information was known to medicine long before the advent of antibiotics. The most accurate microbiological tests for AP were studies of lung tissue in the area of inflammation in deceased patients. The accumulated information on the causative agents of the disease showed that the development of AP is not associated with one specific strain. The probability of the presence of various microorganisms in the focus of inflammation gave reason to reasonably and for many years classify this nosology as acute nonspecific inflammation in the lungs.

In parallel, it was found that AP pathogens can be detected in other parts of the body of healthy people. At the same time, the detection of such microbes in healthy people was not a sign of an impending disease, and such findings were considered as a variant of symbiosis (72). In addition, the lack of historical information about the true epidemics of the disease and any evidence of direct infection in contact with such patients did not allow classifying this nosology as infectious. The assessment of AP as an inflammatory process of nonspecific etiology was based on the totality of the facts that took place and seemed quite reasonable and logical.

Changing views on the role of etiology in the development of AP went in parallel with the use of antibiotics. The introduction of these drugs into clinical practice not only saved millions of human lives, but also laid the foundation for the formation of new problems caused by the negative consequences of this type of treatment. If the initial effectiveness of antibacterial therapy remained the same as in the first years of its use, then there would be no grounds for such a discussion at all. However, it is the decrease in the effectiveness of antibiotics, the increase in the number of resistant strains and the increased role of viruses in the development of AP that are the main reason for the changes that are taking place, which require at least a detailed analysis and objective assessment.

The fact that antibiotics have changed the usual balance between our body and its accompanying microflora is already known not only to specialists with medical education, but also to the general population. New antimicrobials are periodically discussed in the media or problems with stable microflora are mentioned. A retrospective look at the period of antibiotic use allows us to note numerous changes in their arsenal, as well as the appearance and growth of the number of resistant strains. This process from the point of view of the peculiarities of the existence of the biological world was quite expected. On the one hand, the accompanying microflora is a necessary condition for the vital activity of our body, and its complete sterilization is unthinkable even hypothetically. On the other hand, bacteria as living biological objects have the ability to adapt to external influences, which they have convincingly confirmed in response to the aggression of antibiotics.

Contrary to the logic of biological consequences, the formation of new ideas about the role and significance of bacterial pathogens of AP occurred under the strong impression of the effect of the first years of the use of antibiotics and the long-term principles of therapy "antibiotics alone". It was these factors that formed a different idea of the essence of the observed phenomena. If the use of a therapeutic drug with an exclusively antimicrobial effect is enough to make the patient feel better, then this means that the main and in fact the only cause of AP is its causative agent, isn't it? The logic of this conclusion implies considering AP as an infection, and its clinical features as a result of the pathogenic properties of the pathogen.

Looking ahead a bit, it is necessary to mention in this regard one of the unexpected lessons that the SARS-CoV-2 pandemic has taught us. Modern medicine does not have specific remedies against coronavirus, so patients with COVID-19 pneumonia do not receive etiotropic treatment. However, the results of palliative care for coronavirus pneumonia do not actually differ from the general indicators of treatment of patients with CAP, where the latter are provided with antibacterial therapy as the main means of treatment. These statistics, which are presented in more detail in the relevant sections of this book, are a convincing argument against the general excessive demonization of AP pathogens and exaggeration of their role in the genesis and severity of the disease.

2.2.2. Methods for determining the pathogens of AP and their reliability.

If we study the literature on the topic of AP over the past few decades, we will be able to identify individual periods when the era of certain pathogens in the etiology of this disease was proclaimed. Such generalizing conclusions were based not only on an increase in positive bacteriological analyses of one of the pathogens, but also on the impression of changes in the clinical picture of the disease. For example, during the so-called staphylococcal catastrophe, purulent-destructive complications of AP began to be called nothing more than staphylococcal destruction of the lungs. However, when the presence of staphylococcus in the focus of purulent inflammation began to decrease, it became clear that complicated forms of AP of another etiology are almost impossible to distinguish by clinical manifestations from staphylococcal lesions.

The main role in such opinions and assessments was played by the idea that arose with the beginning of the use of antibiotics that the bacterial pathogen of AP is the main cause of its development. The dissemination of this point of view logically required more detailed information about the main causative agents of the disease, but, unfortunately, such information was obtained earlier and continues to be supplemented now mainly by the results of in vitro studies. The comparison of pathogenic properties of individual microorganisms studied in the laboratory was extrapolated to the clinical manifestation of the disease, being the basis for analogies, generalizations and conclusions. The practical application of this information has transformed into the search for the most suitable and effective antimicrobial agents.

To date, the database of bacterial pathogens of AP is quite extensive and detailed, and the list of their main representatives is an integral part of reviews, manuals and monographs on this topic. The main efforts that have been made for many years for the practical implementation of this information have been aimed at the accurate and earliest possible detection of the causative agent in each case of pneumonia. The difficulty of establishing the etiology of AP for many years has served as an explanation for the reasons for the unsuccessful treatment of these patients who were unable to receive targeted use of antibiotics in a timely manner. To solve this problem, a wide variety of methods of direct or indirect presence of certain microorganisms have been used and continue to be used.

In general practice, the actual unavailability of obtaining material directly from the inflammation zone, especially at the very beginning of the disease, caused the determination of microflora in the nasopharynx and oropharynx. The desire to fill in the gaps in the bacteriological rapid diagnosis and to achieve earlier and more accurate antibacterial therapy has led to the fact that this simple testing method was and probably remains one of the most common. The microflora of the upper respiratory tract can be considered the most likely to enter the lung tissue, since this area has a shorter and more direct path to the lesion (73). However, from my point of view, the results of these studies cannot be a reliable confirmation of the etiology of AP, and the simple movement of microorganisms in the direction of the lung tissue is not at all equivalent to the development of inflammation. The doubtfulness of such a mechanism of the disease has been tested in experiments, the results of which are presented below.

The microflora of the nose and oropharynx is very diverse and many healthy people may have conditionally pathogenic microorganisms in its composition, which are classified as pathogens of AP (74). Such a balance between the body and the accompanying microflora can exist indefinitely. However, the presence of these bacteria in the upper respiratory tract is not a sign of an imminent danger of developing inflammation in the lungs. Similarly, the detection of a microbe in the upper respiratory tract is not an absolute proof of its presence in the area of inflammation of the lung tissue.

It should be added to the above that if studies of the microflora of the upper respiratory tract met the requirements of clinicians, there would be no need to use other options and methods of bacteriological diagnosis in patients with AP. However, the methods, even more dubious in their reliability than the previous version, continued to be tested and applied in wide practice.

With the return of the leading position of pneumococcus among the pathogens of AP, bacteriological diagnostics turned into a search for evidence of its presence in the body as a whole. This trend is quite clearly represented by the following quote from Wikipedia. *"Diagnosis is generally made based on clinical suspicion along with a positive culture from a sample from virtually any place in the body"* (75). It should only be clarified that in this case we are not talking about the diagnosis of AP as a whole, but about the bacteriological verification of the diagnosis.

Until now, it was only about standard methods of detecting the microorganism itself. However, in recent years, various methods of indirect determination of the presence in the body, in particular, pneumococcus, have been widely used. Such tests are based on the identification of various types of biomarkers up to the confirmation of urinary antigen (58.76.77). Thus, the goal of bacteriological diagnosis of AP, which should be achieved by identifying the pathogen in the focus of inflammation, eventually transforms into the search for traces of a certain strain in the patient's body. But, in the end, the presence of a certain microbe in the body is not proof of its role in the development of the inflammatory process, is it?

All the variety of microbiological diagnostics of AP has been intensively used and continues to be used only in order to provide targeted antibacterial therapy, the effectiveness of which is constantly decreasing. The results of these long-term efforts have proved fruitless, and in recent years many experts have begun to note as an undoubted fact that the choice of antibiotics in the treatment of AP was and remains empirical. However, these confessions relate only to the definition of the etiology of the process, but did not affect the strategy of solving the problem of AP in any way. The general meaning of such criticism is quite briefly and vividly presented by the following quote. "*The empirical choice of antibacterial therapy is the cornerstone of managing patients with pneumonia. To reduce antibiotic abuse, antibiotic resistance, and side effects, empirical, effective, and individualized treatment with antibiotics is necessary"* (15).

The presented paragraph from the conclusion proposed by the authors of the article very convincingly reflects the widespread efforts today to solve the problem of AP exclusively with the help of etiotropic approaches. The forced statement of the fact that in medical practice the causative agent of pneumonia remains unidentified and antimicrobial therapy is applied on the basis of assumptions, and not the results of bacteriological studies, did not affect the strategy of further decisions. Moreover, it remains completely unclear how the growth of microflora resistance and various side effects of antibiotics can be avoided by continuing their further empirical use.

In addition to the above, it is necessary to add information that is constantly updated and published by the US National Center for Health Statistics and, in particular, its Center for Disease Control and Prevention (78). These reports allow you to find many characteristics of patients who have been treated with a diagnosis of AP. However, there is no information about the etiology of the disease in these summary reports, which is logical and natural, since such accurate statistics do not exist. Moreover, recently, American experts from two leading scientific societies on this issue came to a joint conclusion that efforts to identify pathogens of AP do not affect the results of treatment, and recommend an empirical choice of antibiotics as the basis of treatment (6).

All this information once again makes us pay attention to the fact that many years of efforts to implement a plan for rapid bacteriological diagnosis and targeted antibacterial therapy for each patient with AP have ended in vain. This means that the etiology of the process, which is currently considered as the main cause of the disease, remains unknown in the vast majority of patients. Moreover, if we analyze the totality of various facts about the previous dynamics of AP pathogens over the past decades, hardly anyone will take the liberty to predict the microbial or viral leaders of this process even in the near future.

The assessment of existing approaches to the diagnosis of AP pathogens will be incomplete if we do not pay attention to another variant of their definition, which is not directly related to bacteriological or biomarker methods. This principle of determining the pathogens of AP is a product of the "microbial" concept of the disease and the result of the desire to have at least approximate information about a possible bacterial agent. Initially, attempts were made to determine a possible pathogen based on clinical signs of the disease, but such comparisons and assessments did not bring practical benefits.

One of the most common recent versions of the diagnosis of AP pathogens was based on a comparison of the conditions in which the disease occurred. Various bacteriological studies inside medical institutions, including medical equipment, have shown that more virulent microflora accumulates and concentrates in these conditions. These results are quite logical, since medical institutions are a place of concentration of sick people. Based on these data, differences in the severity of AP depending on the place of its occurrence were considered, which was explained by the participation of various bacterial flora as pathogens of the disease.

The result of this work was the creation of a new classification of acute inflammation in the lungs, depending on the place and conditions of its occurrence (community -acquired, healthcare-associated, hospital-acquired, ventilator-associated etc). The main difference between this gradation of the disease from other variants of classifications was information about the most likely pathogens that are inherent in each form of AP (64,79). This type of testing of patients with AP has become widespread primarily due to its simplicity of application: if necessary, it can be used even when consulting over the phone. It is impossible to judge how much this introduction improved the etiological diagnosis of AP, since the exact results of such testing are unattainable, but, judging by the current results of treatment, there were no significant positive changes.

There is no doubt that the main reasons for the appearance of such an approach, indicating the probable causative agent of AP, was the lack of reliable bacteriological methods of rapid diagnosis and belief in the exceptional role of targeted antibacterial therapy for successful treatment. However, assigning such an important place to the etiological classification of AP cases depending on the localization and conditions of the disease development, the most important feature of the difference between the selected groups of patients was not taken into account.

It is unlikely that anyone will have doubts about the difference between the general condition of a person who continues the normal rhythm of life (community-acquired) and a person who is hospitalized in a hospital (hospital-acquired). The very fact of hospitalization suggests that in the latter case, there are already problems in the body that require correction under the supervision of specialists. If there is inflammation in the lungs against this background, it should be more severe than in a patient who was considered practically healthy at the time of the disease, right?

An even more severe initial condition is typical for patients who need or are already receiving auxiliary ventilation. In the latter case, intubation is an aggravating circumstance in addition to the initial problems. Regardless of the quality of the intubation tube and the skill of the staff, the introduction of a foreign body into the trachea is accompanied by micro-damage to its mucous membrane, and the moment of intubation-the ingress of infected mucus from the oropharynx into its lumen.

Thus, the undoubted difference between these groups is based on the initial state of the patients, which in itself is a sufficient explanation for the different severity of the disease. However, modern gradations of patients with AP do not come from differences in the initial state of the body, but suggest their separation by the nature of the pathogens. This mini-classification is a continuation of the narrow infectious concept of the disease and is widely used in recent years in the analysis of treatment results. At the same time, the totality of various information about the bacteriological diagnosis of AP, published in the literature over the years, indicates the declarative nature of the proposed gradation, but, unfortunately, no one pays attention to this important detail (80,81).

This separation of patients with AP fascinates many with its simplicity of application and is widely used in everyday practice and scientific research. Unfortunately, the artificiality and deceptiveness of such a diagnosis, which, judging by the results of treatment, did not bring obvious practical benefits, remains the most acceptable classification of the disease, the relevance of which will remain as long as its causative agent is considered the main and only cause of the occurrence and development of AP, and its suppression will be considered the main guarantee of therapeutic success.

The concentration of attention on the properties of pathogens remains the dominant trend in research and study of the problem of AP for many years. The narrowness of this approach lies in the fact that an acute inflammatory process in the lungs is one of the examples of conflicts that occur in the biological world. In any conflict, at least two parties involved in the confrontation participate, and each of them contributes its own peculiarity to this process. The development of AP is a conflict between micro- and macroorganism, in which the patient's body is not just a breeding ground for bacteria, but it is another direction in the study of the problem.

It should only be noted here that the priority of the pathogen in the genesis of AP is more declarative, and the disease may have significant differences in the severity of its manifestations in different patients in the presence of one pathogen. This exaggeration, which arose in the process of striving to cure a patient with AP with the help of "antibiotics alone", has no absolute evidence that the bacterial factor determines the fate of these patients. On the contrary, the facts accumulated today point to the important role of various other causes in the emergence and dynamics of this disease.

2.3. Are sepsis and septic shock common complications of AP?

The dominant idea of the leading role of the pathogen in the severity of clinical manifestations of AP suggests a high probability of septic complications of the process in such patients. There is no need to deny the possibility of these complications in the dynamics of AP development, but it is impossible to ignore the fact that in recent years the severity of the condition of such patients is considered almost exclusively as a result of the development of sepsis and septic shock in them. Such interpretations of septic complications of AP would not cause doubts and reasonable objections if they had objective confirmations, and not assumptions based on analogies with other diseases.

Bacterial sepsis and septic shock have for many years been considered the most severe complications and the main cause of death in patients with AP. Over the past couple of years, the number of patients with viral pneumonia has increased dramatically, but the frequency of septic complications among them, no longer bacterial, but viral etiology, actually remains the same (82-84). The simplicity of determining the septic nature of these complications, which has no microbiological confirmation in the overwhelming number of observations, should raise doubts about the validity of such statements, since the diagnosis sets the direction of therapeutic efforts and determines the final result.

According to the old classifications, the peculiarity of the body's reaction to the inflammatory process was considered in the form of three main forms of manifestation of its reactivity: hypoergic, normoergic and hyperergic. That is, such a gradation divided one of the main characteristics of inflammatory diseases into possible variants from cases with a relatively slow and not always noticeable course of the process to the most aggressive and lightning-fast forms.

In recent years, the interpretation of the clinical manifestations of AP and its septic complications has been based on the concept of systemic inflammatory response syndrome (SIRS) with indication of its clinical and laboratory criteria (25,85,86). At the same time, experts in their assessments believe that in previous definitions of sepsis and septic shock, excessive attention was paid to the process of inflammation, while the sensitivity of SIRS parameters for the diagnosis of septic complications is not specific enough.

As a result, an important place in the definition of sepsis is given to the Sequential (Sepsis-related) Organ Failure Assessment (SOFA). With this method of determining the diagnosis, the etiology of complications is not a determining parameter, but the clinical consequences of the main process play a decisive role (25,85). Objective criteria that could confirm that this clinical situation is due to the generalization of infection, and no other mechanisms, are not decisive in this approach to determining the diagnosis.

In the modern interpretation, the concept of SIRS in AP combines reactions of the body that do not have the character of severe manifestations. According to the proposed criteria, such a group may include both relatively mild and moderate forms of the disease, when moderate deviations of the respiratory and cardiovascular systems are recorded, but no other violations are observed.

In case of signs of organ dysfunction, the condition of patients and the nature of complications are determined based on SOFA using points. If 2 or more points are obtained during the analysis of indicators, then this situation is regarded as sepsis. If there are particularly deep disorders of blood circulation and metabolic processes, then we are already talking about septic shock.

Such a diagnosis looks quite simple and easily doable compared to the previous criteria. For example, there is no need for mandatory microbiological confirmation of these complications as septic, and diagnoses of "sepsis" or "septic shock" themselves are an early explanation for very likely treatment failures, since mortality with the development of these conditions increases sharply (85). At the same time, it should be noted that the very concept of septic complications has undergone drastic changes, and no one wonders to what extent the described criteria correspond to and are due to the generalization of infection.

In the literature on this issue, only isolated reports of bacterial forms of AP can be found, in which the frequency of detection of bacteria in the blood of patients with this disease is only from 10.7% to 12%, including not only cases of sepsis and septic shock, but also bacteremia (87,88). Even in patients with septic shock, the frequency of positive blood cultures is only from 13.2% to 18%, and the comparative mortality rates from this complication of AP among patients with positive and negative tests have no significant differences (76,89).

The idea of the causes of the severity of clinical manifestations of AP should change dramatically if we recall the fundamental features of lung tissue damage. Modern publications do not pay due attention to the peculiarities of the mechanisms accompanying inflammation in the lungs, therefore, cases of sepsis and septic shock in patients with AP are analyzed in the general group of similar complications in other diseases. The general material of the analysis of these complications usually includes information about diseases of various localization with cardinal differences in pathogenesis, where patients with lung tissue inflammation account for up to 40-50% (25). This confusion of material is a very serious misconception about such analytical work.

Even very scant information on the topic covered, which is presented above, gives reason for reflection and a thorough analysis of the validity of existing ideas. Such an examination will not bring full-fledged conclusions if we ignore a number of fundamental foundations of the AP. First of all, it is necessary to recall the general mechanisms of inflammatory transformation of tissues in the affected area.

There is no need to prove the fact that the basis of the pathological restructuring of tissue structures in the focus of acute inflammation is the indispensable development of a consistent reaction of blood vessels with a violation of blood flow in them and increased permeability of the walls. This transformation is also necessarily accompanied by five classic signs of inflammation: heat, pain, redness, swelling and loss of function (90). The last sign, a violation of the function of the affected organ, plays a leading role in the clinical manifestations and features of the disease.

But, the main feature of the topic under discussion is the fact that AP is the only inflammatory process that occurs in the small circle of blood circulation, unlike all other nosologies localized in the large circle. The inverse proportion of the functional state between the two circulatory circles with their inseparable anatomical and functional connection and interdependence underlies the fundamental differences between the pathological mechanisms of AP and inflammatory diseases of other localization. In this regard, the interpretation of the pathogenesis of AP by analogy with other forms of acute inflammation can in no way have the same scenario. The assessment of the detected deviations of blood flow parameters should also have a different interpretation.

The volume of blood that is released by the left ventricle of the heart into the large circle of blood circulation should be absolutely equal to its volume, which enters the vessels of the lungs. This strict rule of normal blood circulation and vital activity of the body is supported by a significantly lower pressure in the vessels of the small circle of blood circulation. Violation of this balance leads to functional disorders in the cardiovascular system ,and in order to correct the imbalance, if it occurs, we do not need to look for suitable ways to correct it. In our body, there are various natural mechanisms that are aimed at automatically correcting a dangerous situation.

One of these mechanisms was discovered and described in the thirties of the last century by Schwiegk (91). We are talking about a reflex on the part of the baroreceptors of the pulmonary vessels, which is triggered in the event of an increase in blood pressure in them. Physiologists, in accordance with the action of this mechanism, often call it the unloading reflex. Thus, increased pressure in the pulmonary vessels leads to a reflex decrease in systemic arterial pressure and, in particular, to an increase in blood supply to the spleen and vasodilation in skeletal muscles. The expansion of peripheral vessels reduces blood flow to the small circulatory circle and, consequently, unloads the pulmonary capillaries and protects the lungs from edema.

The appearance of a focus of acute inflammation in the vessels of the small circle is a disaster for the body and a cause that disrupts the balance between the two halves of the circulatory system. Localization of this zone not only creates a physical obstacle to the main blood flow, which is ejected by the right half of the heart (figure 2), but also is a source of reflex spasm of the pulmonary vessels (91-93). The capacity of the small circle decreases, while the pressure in its vessels begins to increase. In order to correct this situation and avoid asynchronous operation of the cardiovascular system, incompatible with life, the body changes the parameters of a large circle of blood circulation, reducing the pressure in it and increasing its volume for a sudden "excess" of circulating blood (Schwiegk's reflex).

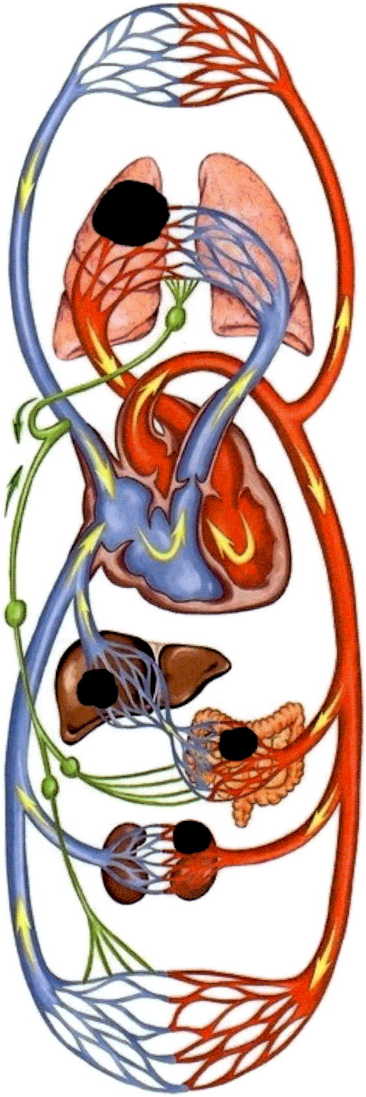

Figure 2. Schematic representation of the human circulatory system. The comparative significance of foci of acute inflammation (black fields) in different organs and their effect on the blood flow, depending on the possible localization.

The presented scheme clearly shows that the focus of inflammation in the lung always lies in the path of the general main blood flow, reducing the possibility of free movement of the entire volume of circulating blood. In this case, we are talking about a purely physical obstacle, which is further enhanced by the inclusion of reflex and humoral factors. At the same time, the focus of inflammation in the large circle of blood circulation, regardless of localization, initially affects only the parameters of the corresponding regional blood flow. In other words, the localization of inflammation in the zone of the small circulatory circle itself creates prerequisites for generalized blood flow disorders identical to the signs of septic complications, while peripheral foci lead to such deviations at later stages of the disease as a result of generalization of infection.

The described mechanism of regulation of blood flow in the event of a catastrophe in the small circle of blood circulation is actually more complex, since humoral factors, including hormones, also take part in it. For example, it is well known about the renin–angiotensin–aldosterone system (RAAS), which is a chain of regulation of blood flow and in which the lungs are directly involved (94). However, in this context, we are not talking about the details of this biological phenomenon, but about its essence, which is that it performs its task automatically, trying to restore the necessary proportions to the circulatory system between its two contours and preserve its functionality.

Autonomous regulation of blood circulation is one of the fundamental biological laws of our life. No one feels any changes in the ratios between the indicators of the two circulatory circles, which constantly arise in the process of vital activity and changing situations, but are aligned automatically without our conscious efforts. Alarms arise in our consciousness only when the adaptive capabilities of the body have reached their limits and the body receives a warning about the existing danger. The affected subject begins to feel a lack of air, weakness, dizziness and other disturbing sensations. Examination of such patients makes it possible to note an increase in respiration and pulse, a decrease in blood pressure and other deviations from the initial indicators of the vital activity of the body.

The described mechanism of redistribution of circulating blood in the case of changes in blood pressure in the pulmonary vessels allows the body to avoid hemodynamic shifts that become incompatible with life. The more aggressively the inflammatory process develops, the less time the body has to adapt and the more serious deviations are observed as a result. The range of possible clinical options for the development of AP suggests the likelihood of rapid deterioration of the condition of these patients, when with the lightning-fast development of the inflammatory process, hemodynamic disorders reach critical situations. Currently, such conditions are regarded as sepsis or septic shock, although we are talking about different degrees of manifestation of the same mechanism.

The rate of dynamics of the inflammatory process in the lung tissue, even in the case of the most lightning-fast forms, is in no way comparable with the development of pulmonary embolism (PE), the reflex mechanism of which is almost identical to a similar reaction in AP. And although the clinical manifestations of this pathology can vary from an asymptomatic picture to sudden death, it is the instant and abrupt appearance of severe symptoms that arouses interest in the causes of this pathology (95-99). In the most severe case, a clinical picture of shock with abnormally low blood pressure and sudden death is almost immediately observed (100). With all the variety of consequences of PE, it was noted that its clinical manifestations do not directly depend on the size of the embolus, which indicates differences in the individual response of the body to an equivalent stimulus.

The presented small comparison of AP with PE allows us to look at the problem discussed in this section from a slightly different point of view. Firstly, both in the case of inflammation and as a result of embolus administration, the primary link in the entire subsequent chain of pathophysiological transformations is the wall of the pulmonary vessels. Secondly, the inextricable link between morphology and function indicates the inevitability of identical functional deviations, since we are talking about the impact on the same morphological structure. Finally, despite the identity between the description of the clinical picture of shock in PE and the so-called septic shock in AP, the first of them, as a rule, does not have a septic nature.

An exception to the standard pathogenesis and clinical picture of PE is the hematogenic introduction of infected emboli into the lungs. But then we are talking about a completely different disease. After all, in such a situation there is always a focus of purulent inflammation on the periphery, the ingress of infected emboli into the vessels of the small circulatory circle indicates the generalization of infection, and the observed complication is the beginning of the septic form of AP, which in this case is a secondary process in the body, isn't it?

The modern interpretation of the most severe manifestations of AP as a result of septic complications is based solely on the recognition of the dominant role of the pathogen in this disease. When forming this concept, the uniqueness of emerging pathological mechanisms that radically distinguish AP from other inflammatory processes is not taken into account. This approach creates all further ideas about the nature of this disease and directs subsequent diagnostic and therapeutic actions exclusively by analogy with other localizations of inflammation. The deepening of these misconceptions is clearly manifested in the choice of principles for assessing the condition of patients.

The idea of septic complications of AP today involves diagnosis, interpretation and their subsequent correction based on the parameters of peripheral blood flow. These principles, on which the assessment of the condition of patients with other localizations of the primary focus of inflammation is based, have the opposite meaning in patients with AP, when shifts in systemic circulation are secondary and more reflect the adaptation process than direct manifestations of the disease. In this regard, it is not superfluous to recall that the pressure in the pulmonary vessels is significantly inferior to this indicator on the periphery, which under normal conditions exceeds it by 5-8 times (101).

The current situation with the diagnosis and treatment of AP complications is quite paradoxical. On the one hand, recommendations and protocols in this direction are focused on the leading role of the etiological factor in the development and course of the disease. On the other hand, the existing principles allow the free use of such diagnoses as "sepsis" and "septic shock", only on the basis of clinical and laboratory, and not bacteriological data.

The strangeness and inconsistency of such a situation is emphasized by the fact that such odious diagnoses as sepsis and septic shock do not require their basic confirmation, but the modern ideology of the AP provides an appropriate explanation for this case. Expert assessments take into account the absence of pathogenic microorganisms in the bloodstream as a result of preliminary antibacterial therapy (102-104). Such conclusions look even more strange, since it is claimed that highly effective antimicrobial therapy could not protect the patient from generalization of infection, and the pathogen itself is absent. By the way, some experts have drawn attention to the fact that negative microbiological tests in patients with sepsis are usually detected in cases where the cause of this complication is AP, but do not provide an explanation for this feature (104,105).

The ideology of this misconception continues to spread today to COVID-19 pneumonia. The severity of this form of the disease is explained by the development of viral sepsis and viral shock, which are considered as the causes of negative dynamics in patients only by analogy with the existing concept of AP (82,83). There are no objective confirmations and even attempts to objectively diagnose these viral complications. H.C. Prescott and T.D. Girard (84), analyzing the features of COVID-19 pneumonia among hospitalized patients, frankly note that viral sepsis in them resembles (!) bacterial and develops in 20% of these observations, but they also do not confirm these figures with any microbiological arguments.

In conclusion of this section, it should be noted that AP, regardless of its causative agent, is one nosological form, which is based on inflammatory damage to the same morphological structures with a violation of their function. The development of pathological changes occurs according to one scenario, which has individual differences with the variants of the speed and depth of damage. The designation of these phenomena as SIRS, immune response, individual reactivity of the body or other terms does not change the essence of the processes taking place. Generalization of infection is quite acceptable in this variant of the inflammatory process, but it can only worsen the situation, not being the main cause of a severe AP clinic.

2.4. Are etiotropic drugs the main method of treatment of acute pneumonia?

In the middle of the last century, a significant event took place in medicine, the biological role and didactic significance of which have not yet been fully realized. We are talking about the discovery and the beginning of the use of antibiotics, which changed not only the basic principles of the treatment of inflammatory processes, but also had a specific impact on the formation of professional ideas in some areas of medicine. The first experience of treating many severe inflammatory diseases with antibiotics has brought fantastic results that could not even have been expected before. These drugs have saved millions of lives, and despite the loss of their initial effectiveness, they continue to retain their therapeutic value with reasonable and rational use.

Antibiotics are still one of the most popular medicines. At the same time, a fifth (19%) of antibiotic prescriptions to patients are due to pneumonia (52). Their action, unlike other representatives of the pharmacopoeia, is directed not at the structures and substances of the body, but at its microflora. The action of antibiotics cannot be directed only against the suspected pathogens of AP. Their introduction into the body affects those representatives of the microflora who turned out to be sensitive to this drug. In this regard, antimicrobial treatment can create broad biological side effects. It is impossible to avoid such results of antibacterial therapy, and their stability and prevalence with the further use of antibiotics retain the prerequisites for strengthening these negative consequences. These features underlie many non-standard phenomena and actions that are associated with the use of antibiotics.

Firstly, each representative of the microbial world is in itself a separate biological object with the ability to adapt to new conditions. As a result of prolonged exposure to antibiotics on the accompanying microflora of the body, a whole galaxy of resistant strains has appeared.

Secondly, the continuing increase in the number of varieties of resistant strains and their number does not bear signs of an epidemiological problem, but in the case of a disease, the difficulties of therapeutic tasks and the forced need for the constant creation of more effective antimicrobials increase. So, almost 10 years ago, the detection rate of MRSA alone in patients with community-acquired pneumonia ranged from 3.3% to 7.6% (106).

Thirdly, the exclusively antimicrobial effect of antibiotics is an explanation for the fact that the same drug can be used as a general therapeutic agent for diseases that are completely incomparable with each other. In addition, it should be borne in mind that with such a therapeutic effect, the elimination of functional and morphological disorders that do not disappear instantly when the bacterial factor of inflammation is suppressed depends on the capabilities of the organism itself.

Today, the discussion of antibiotic-resistant strains of pathogens, the list of which has appeared in recent decades and continues to grow, has become commonplace. The detection of such strains in healthy people when tested during routine medical examinations is no longer considered an emergency. Dysbiosis has also become a habitual probability of long-term antimicrobial treatment.

During the period of widespread use of antibiotics, a change of leaders among AP pathogens began to be observed. In the pre-antibiotic period, this disease rightfully belonged to polyethological and nonspecific, although the leading role in its etiology was attributed to pneumococcus. In the literature, it was not possible to find special studies confirming the effect of this therapy on the dynamics of the etiology of the disease, however, this phenomenon, which in the past was not so obvious, is quite consistent with the side effect of antibiotics. For example, an analysis of materials obtained in dynamics over the past few years from 890 hospitals in the United States showed that the antibiotic-resistant microflora continues to grow, and the proportion and prevalence of individual strains among the total number of such observations are constantly changing (107). Prolonged suppression of one type of AP pathogens leads to a gradual predominance of other microorganisms in the development of this process. This phenomenon of recent decades is just another indirect proof that the causes of the disease do not directly depend on the variants of microflora.

To the above, it is necessary to add such an undoubted statistical fact as the steady increase in the incidence of AP of viral etiology, which has been observed in recent decades (11-13). The shift in the etiology of lung inflammation towards viral forms is another result of the long-term suppression of the microbial segment of our microbiological support. This postulate cannot be accepted as an absolute argument, but further developments should show the trends existing in this section. In the meantime, it can be stated that over the past couple of decades, the coronavirus epidemics have turned into a pandemic, and vaccinations do not give full guarantees and require their repetition due to the appearance of more and more new strains. This picture suggests that humanity is entering the era of viral diseases. If the future begins to confirm these gloomy assumptions, then their results should be considered as a side effect of our achievements and efforts in the field of antimicrobial therapy.

For example, currently the results of comparison and search for the most optimal antibiotic in patients with community-acquired pneumonia continue to be published, although data on the etiology of the disease remain inconclusive, and the number of viral lesions among them is unknown (63,108). The material obtained does not allow the authors of these publications to draw a concrete conclusion from the work, which, from my point of view, is quite natural, but they emphasize the need to continue such research. The latest recommendations illustrate the depth and stability of views that have developed under the auspices of an uncritical belief in the exclusivity of antibiotics.

The peculiarities of antibiotics that have only an antibacterial effect and do not affect the vital links of pathogenesis do not allow us to consider them as the leading and even more so the only means of treating AP. But for many years, the bulk of these patients were treated on the principle of "antibiotics alone", isn't it? If we add to this the above-mentioned side effects of this method, then the further use of drugs of this group should be carried out under much stricter control than it is being carried out now. However, in this situation, an insurmountable obstacle arises, due to many years of didactic traditions. Medical training based on the expected benefits of antimicrobial principles today orients therapeutic efforts in the same direction, despite changing conditions with a loss of logic and meaning.

At the moment, the recommendations of specialists and specific approaches to treatment demonstrate a subconscious desire to preserve old stereotypes, despite the change in the etiology of AP and the inadequacy of antibacterial therapy to new conditions. The appearance of a large number of patients with COVID-19 pneumonia led to the fact that antibiotics that do not have an antiviral effect automatically lost their purpose. However, this logical reassessment does not correspond to the real state of affairs.

Currently, in patients hospitalized with COVID-19 pneumonia, bacterial infection is detected only in a small number of observations. The accuracy of the methods for determining bacterial pathogens of AP has long raised great doubts about their reliability, but if we take into account the published results, coronavirus inflammation of the lung tissue is combined with the layering of the bacterial component in 7-8% of cases (109, 110). In other studies, this result increased to 20.9% as a result of the use of various tests, including serology, urine analysis for antigen, nasopharyngeal smears (111). But even the latest figures are significantly lower than the number of patients with COVID-19 who receive antibiotics.

Despite the lack of direct indications for the appointment of antimicrobials, the coverage of this type of treatment for COVID-19 pneumonia is impressive. During the pandemic, these patients continue to receive antibiotics in 70-80 percent or more of cases (109,111-115). Most of these decisions do not have direct confirmation of such a need. It is considered sufficient to prescribe antibiotics if the patient has evidence of the inflammatory nature of the process in the lungs: the clinical picture, some laboratory data, X-ray diagnostics (113). Additional incentives for this therapy may be prolonged hypoxia, the need for hardware support, advanced age, concomitant diseases (110). That is, in the presence of viral pneumonia, antibiotics remain in the role of a treatment familiar to the attending physicians, and not a means of treatment that new patients need.

A number of authors are trying to substantiate and prove the need to preserve the previous approaches to antibacterial therapy regardless of the viral etiology of the disease (116). While maintaining the inviolability of old stereotypes of medical care, some healthcare systems automatically include patients with coronavirus infection in the treatment regimen for community-acquired pneumonia (117,118). However, it's no secret that such treatment regimens are based primarily on the leading role of antibiotics.

The described difficulties in implementing targeted antimicrobial therapy have long been the reason for the lengthening of treatment courses, but in recent years there have been recommendations and relevant clinical experience in patients with AP using short (within 3-5 days) courses of antibiotics (6,119-121). For many it turned out to be unexpected and inexplicable that such a sharp reduction in the timing of antibiotic prescribing did not affect the results of treatment. From my point of view, this information is another argument in favor of the previous statement that antibiotics do not decide the fate of such patients and it is necessary to take into account other circumstances affecting the dynamics of the inflammatory process in the lungs.

The emergence of the SARS-CoV-2 pandemic has significantly changed the working conditions of emergency medical services. The rapid spread of the coronavirus has led to the need for strict compliance with epidemiological measures, which are strictly carried out at the planetary level. However, these measures cannot fully solve the problems that have arisen due to the sharp increase in the flow of patients with viral pneumonia. This situation is similar to a kind of test for checking medicine, where wildlife acts as an examiner. Such a turn of events requires brainstorming to solve it with a detailed analysis of all the information related to this problem. However, the real state of affairs in this direction shows that the principles of the approach to acute inflammation of the lung tissue, learned over many years, dominate the interpretation of the problem and its solution.

If with bacterial forms of AP with a long list of possible pathogens, one of the main reasons for treatment failures was considered the difficulty of choosing targeted antibacterial therapy, now we are talking about monoethology, but the failures are explained by the lack of effective etiotropic drugs. Under these conditions, the preservation of the previous strategy with an emphasis on the leading role of the AP pathogen and the decisive importance of its suppression is clearly manifested. This ideology is reflected in the intensified search for drugs that would act on the coronavirus with the same success as antibiotics affect bacteria, but the endless stream of publications on this topic still boils down to one conclusion that no such drugs have been found (122).

The versatile efforts that are being made to suppress viruses and achieve tangible results in seriously ill patients remain fruitless. Virus neutralization is usually demonstrated in laboratory studies when the tested drug is in direct contact with the object (475-477). However, in the real conditions of a living organism, the laboratory effect of such attempts is not achieved, which has its own logical reasons and explanations, which are not always given importance.

First of all, it is well known that clinical signs of viral pneumonia appear during the period of the disease when the pathogen is already inside the cell. In such a situation, drugs that can affect the virus in the laboratory are not always able to follow the pathogen into the cell, and when they have this ability, they can aggravate the toxic effect on cellular structures (475).

In addition, suppressing the pathogen at a time when the patient needs urgent care due to an increasing cascade of severe functional disorders is a belated measure. At this stage of the disease, the pathogen does not determine the intensity and severity of clinical manifestations, which was noted when attempting differential diagnosis of AP on an etiological basis. For example, long-term attempts to separate bacterial forms of the disease by the nature of the pathogen ultimately had no effect on clinical symptoms and further treatment results (6,15).

The monopoly of old ideas on the problem of AP in new conditions continues to lead researchers in the same narrow direction, forcing them to recheck the stages already passed. For example, the antibiotic "azithromycin" has been used in medicine for more than 30 years not only for bacterial forms of AP, but also for inflammation of the middle ear, streptococcal pharyngitis and even diarrhea (123). Currently, this drug, which has no proven antiviral activity, is undergoing clinical trials against coronavirus (124). This choice for the search can only be explained by the lack of other ideas to solve the problem, but the preservation of existing views on the problem highlights the fact that, having received no evidence of a positive effect of this antibiotic against coronavirus, the authors propose to continue this study. The meaning of such a sentence is unclear, as if additional testing could bring the exact opposite result?

Thus, antibiotics, even in the initial period of their maximum effectiveness, were not a specific means of helping with AP and cannot correspond to the concept of the main, and even more so the only method of treating this disease. To date, the long-term use of antibiotics has reached a period when the preservation of their effectiveness can no longer be supported only by the development of new-generation drugs. The side effects of antibacterial therapy continue to change the microbiological environment around us. One of the consequences of this type of treatment is the growing tendency to change the pathogens of AP with the growth of viral forms of the disease and a decrease in the role of antimicrobials themselves.

During the presentation of this section, quite a lot of information was presented that in addition to the biological consequences that have been actively discussed for a long time, the long-term use of antibiotics has created another problem that remains hidden, despite its seriousness and fundamental nature. In this case, we are talking about the didactic influence of this therapeutic direction on the formation of narrow conceptual views on the solution of this problem. The current ideology of the AP today is an obstacle, without the elimination of which it is unthinkable to achieve tangible success in solving the problem under discussion.

The biological consequences of the widespread use of antibiotics have already passed the point of no return, and they should be perceived as a persistent phenomenon that can develop further. This point of view is not isolated, and similar concerns can already be found in current publications (110). However, in order to understand the depth and significance of these consequences for the future, as well as to neutralize the observed trends, it is necessary to realize the didactic negative impact of this type of therapy on the formation of a professional worldview. This is the only consequence of antibiotics that can be corrected, and its correction depends entirely on each of us.

2.5. Do patients with acute pneumonia need intravenous infusions?

Currently, almost all urgently hospitalized patients immediately get access to the venous bed and begin to receive an infusion of solutions. This priority of this procedure is due not only to the need to have the most effective way of administering medications, but also to compensate for the loss of fluid, which in acute diseases has many reasons for this. Further recommendations for the correction of water-electrolyte and volume losses and the choice of the infusion rate are determined by the general criteria for their diagnosis in accordance with the parameters of the large circle of blood circulation. Considering AP, first of all, as a result of infection and not focusing on the localization of the process, modern medicine does not make exceptions in this therapeutic direction for patients with inflammation of the lung tissue.

For many years, fever and tachypnea were considered the main causes of fluid deficiency in patients with AP (39). But the role of these factors in the occurrence of inconspicuous losses is hardly worthy of comparison with the consequences of homeostasis disorders accompanying such diseases as, for example, enterocolitis or peritonitis, when the body really loses large volumes of fluid. Such losses are very noticeable and can be estimated both quantitatively and qualitatively.

Try to compare the volume and quality of losses through the gastrointestinal tract that occur as a result of repeated vomiting and diarrhea, as well as intense exudate into the intestinal lumen and into the abdominal cavity with peritonitis, with the evaporation of fluid during breathing and an increase in body temperature. Even if we imagine that in all patients with AP during hospitalization, the respiratory rate is twice higher than normal, and the body temperature is stable at 38-39 degrees Celsius, the approximate loss of fluid from the body as a result of increased evaporation will not be able to approach the volume and quality of the above emissions. Nevertheless, all patients with a severe and aggressive course of the disease, regardless of the localization of the focus of inflammation, are recommended to inject fluid with boluses (25,82,86,105,125).

Latent fluid loss in patients with AP is described as one of the causes of circulatory disorders, and dehydration as a result of increased evaporation considere a serious problem even at the very beginning of the disease, which raises even greater doubts, since the reason for this conclusion may be a tendency to hypotension or simply analogies with hemodynamic disorders in other similar observations. Usually this explanation is the reason for the appointment of infusions with an uncomplicated course of the disease immediately at the time of hospitalization of the patient in the hospital. Despite the unlikely role of evaporation mechanisms in the development of severe circulatory disorders in AP, the registration of hypotension, as well as sepsis and septic shock (in modern interpretation) in these patients are considered an important cause of immediate infusions (25,82, 86,105,125).

The reasons leading to the rapid appearance of signs of hypotension in patients with AP without visible large fluid losses were discussed above. Here it is only necessary to emphasize once again that the assessment of hemodynamic disorders in patients of this group is based on the parameters of peripheral blood circulation, while their cause and primary shifts in the circulatory system are in the vessels of the small circle. To date, special sets of tests have been proposed that are used to assess the severity of patients' condition. These principles are used in patients regardless of the underlying disease, including AP.

Among the most common methods of assessing the condition of patients, the following can be noted: APACHE II (Acute physiology and chronic health assessment II), CURB-65 (confusion, urea, respiratory rate, blood pressure, age ⩾ 65 years), PSI, the method of determining which is not much different from the first method (126-129). If we compare these assessment methods, it can be noted that the registration of peripheral blood pressure is the leading characteristic of circulatory disorders. However, it should be noted that the value of this indicator and its interpretation remain equivalent for all possible diseases and there are no exceptions for AP.

The use of these testing systems distributes all observations according to severity, when patients with different and incomparable diseases receive equivalent scores. Thus, patients with pneumonia can receive the same characteristics of their condition as patients with diarrhea or peritonitis, and in accordance with treatment protocols, they will receive supportive and intensive therapy on a par with the latter.

Such an assessment system is simple enough for practical application. This makes it possible to unify the general results of deviations of vital signs in patients with various pathologies and, depending on the final result, to systematize and conduct standard intensive therapy. The introduction of these principles into clinical practice facilitates and standardizes the work of attending physicians, as well as guarantees patients the necessary amount of medical care, which was determined by leading specialists. The only group of patients who, from my point of view, do not benefit as a result of such innovations are patients with AP.

A vulnerable feature of these methods, popular in intensive care units, for determining the severity of the condition and prognosis of patients is that they do not reflect differences in diagnoses and localization of the underlying process. Such generalization of various diseases and interpretation of disorders in the light of one standard pathogenesis is the main drawback in the assessment of patients with AP. According to these assessment systems, patients with AP should receive infusion therapy when the first signs of hypotension are detected. If this sign continues to progress, then, in accordance with existing ideas about the leading role of the pathogen in this process, the speed and volume of intravenous infusions begin to increase, since such situations are already regarded as sepsis or septic shock.

In order to pay attention to the features of AP, which are important in the case of intravenous infusions for these patients, it is necessary to list the most significant of them again.

Firstly, inflammation of the lung tissue remains the only disease among such processes that occurs in the small circle of blood circulation.

Secondly, the synchronicity of the work of the two halves of the cardiovascular system is ensured by the entry of equal volumes of blood into them and significantly lower pressure in the pulmonary vessels.

Thirdly, the violation of parity between the small and large circles of blood circulation is incompatible with life, and functional deviations that constantly occur both in the process of vital activity of the body and in the case of diseases are leveled by the autonomous regulatory system (91).

Fourth, the inflammatory transformation of tissues is based on a sequential step-by-step reaction of blood vessels in the affected area with impaired blood flow and a sharp increase in the permeability of the vascular wall. In the lung tissue devoid of pain receptors, the protective role is played by the baroreceptors of the pulmonary vessels, which contribute to a reflex decrease in their throughput (91.93), saving the lungs from overload and edema.

Finally, an acute inflammatory process is inevitably accompanied by five classic signs described many centuries ago by Celsus and Galen and received indisputable confirmation on the basis of subsequent medical experience: heat, pain, redness, swelling, and loss of function. Therefore, these factors will act independently of our attitude to them, and the violation of function will determine the features of the clinic of the disease, depending on the affected organ.

If we now take into account the information presented, then the functional consequences of inflammation in the small circle of blood circulation begin to radically differ from similar processes of peripheral localization. Attention has already been drawn to the fact that a sudden lesion of the lung tissue prevents the circulation of the general blood flow, while other localizations of inflammation are accompanied by circulatory disorders in regional segments of the vascular network. Localization of the focus of inflammation in the small circle is also of particular importance in the case of infusion therapy. The following diagram can give a visual representation of the direction of infusion solutions in the vascular system of the body (Fig. 3).

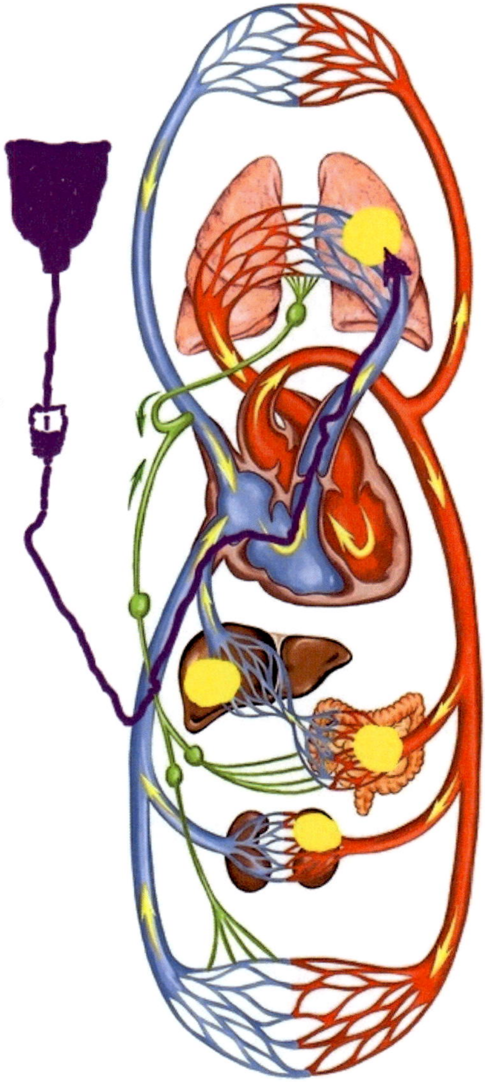

Figure 3. Schematic representation of the human circulatory system. The initial route of intravenous administration of solutions is shown (dark purple arrow) relative to the foci of acute inflammation (yellow fields), depending on the localization.

The influence of the focus of inflammation in the lung on the blood flow in the small circle of circulation is much more complicated than just a physical obstacle. The regulation of synchronicity between the two circulatory circles works independently of our desires at the slightest shifts. It has been known for almost a century about the presence of baroreceptors in the pulmonary vessels, the irritation of which is accompanied by their spasm and a decrease in pressure in the peripheral vessels of the large circle (91). This reflex mechanism, known in the medical literature as the discharge reflex, is our salvation in case of unforeseen circumstances that have arisen in the vascular pool of the lungs.

With AP, as a result of changes in the structure and function of the pulmonary vessels, a relative excess of venous return occurs, and the body seeks to eliminate this dangerous disorder that threatens pulmonary edema. The more intensively the inflammatory process develops, the more difficult it is for the body to compensate for these shifts in blood circulation. Examination of such a patient usually reveals a decrease in blood pressure at the periphery, which serves as the basis for intravenous infusions. The lack of the expected effect is the reason for the increase in the infusion rate. As a result, a paradox arises, a more detailed analysis of which can clarify some features of the dynamics of the AP.

The paradox of this situation is that, on the one hand, the body makes efforts to relieve the small circle of blood circulation. One of the manifestations of such adaptation are signs of hypotension. On the other hand, a decrease in blood pressure in the periphery is considered as a consequence of septic complications, which, according to the dominant recommendations, requires intravenous infusions. Intravenous administration of solutions increases venous inflow and disrupts adaptive mechanisms. In addition to the anticompensatory nature of such therapy, it has another negative quality in the initial period of AP. The first tissue barrier that the injected solutions reach includes a zone of increasing inflammatory edema and infiltration (Fig. 3).

The need to clarify the role of infusion therapy in the dynamics of the development of lung inflammation arose in our work many years ago, when the most aggressive bacterial forms of AP began to be purposefully hospitalized in our department during the initial period of the disease. The concentration of a large number of such patients was accompanied by the rapid development of pleural complications and high mortality in them. To find out the causes of this phenomenon, special studies were conducted. The results obtained are presented below in the relevant sections. Here is also one of the typical examples of our observations of such a development of events.

A 2-year-old girl was taken to the clinic with abdominal pain and shortness of breath 12 hours after their appearance. According to her medical history, the child was healthy, but in the last few days she had a mild respiratory syndrome with a runny nose and a cough without fever. Upon admission to the clinic, the patient was diagnosed with AP (Fig. 4). Intensive treatment was immediately started, including intravenous administration of two antibiotics and intravenous fluids up to 30 ml / kg / hour for 2 hours, followed by a decrease in the infusion rate to 10 ml/ kg/ hour. Despite the treatment, the child's condition did not improve, and a control radiograph was diagnosed with pyopneumothorax 36 hours after hospitalization (Fig. 5). The pus obtained from the pleural cavity during drainage was subjected to bacteriological and microscopic examination, but no microflora was found in it.

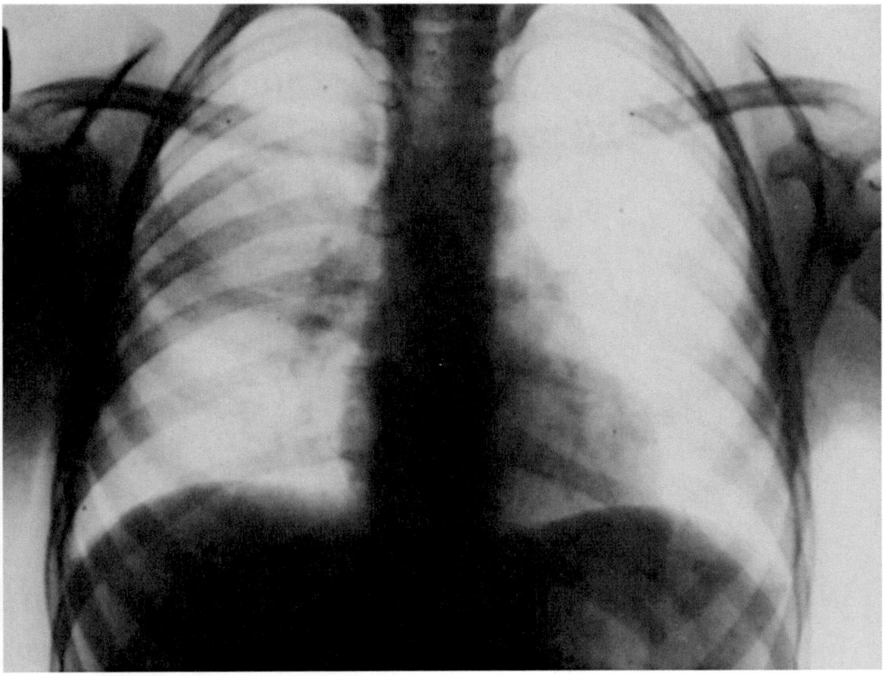

Figure 4. X-ray photograph of 2 y.o. girl 12 hours after the first signs of AP with abdominal pain syndrome were discovered. There is homogeneous shading in a middle-right pulmonary field.

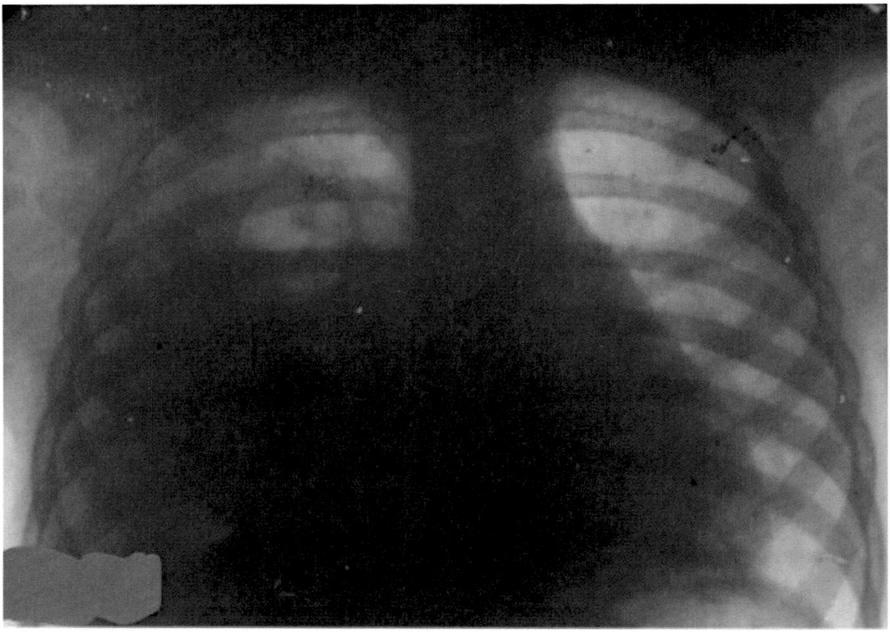

Figure 5. X-ray of the same patient (see Fig. 4), 36 hours after the start of inpatient treatment. There is an intense uniform darkening of almost the entire right lung with a cavity and fluid level in the upper pulmonary field and with a displacement of the mediastinum to the left.

The features of the presented observation allow us to note the extreme aggressiveness of the development of the inflammatory process in the right lung, which in a relatively short period of time reached the stage of severe complications. The time interval between the first and second chest radiographs was only 36 hours. I think many experts will recall similar observations from their own practice. Usually, this course of events is considered to be the result of high virulence of the pathogen, but in this case, the study of pus from the pleural cavity did not confirm this hypothesis.

The case description presented cannot be an absolute proof of the negative effect of infusion therapy on the dynamics of the inflammatory process in the lungs. The results of the observed transformation in the area of inflammation only allow us to assume such a dependence and draw appropriate conclusions based on a number of observations. However, even such an analysis gives grounds to investigate other (besides infection) causes of parapneumonic effusion, the frequency of which in community-acquired pneumonia continues to reach 20-50% of cases, and pleural empyema can be sterile in microbiological studies (130). Today, treatment stereotypes, including intravenous infusions of this category of patients, continue to dominate in a wide world practice, and the statistics of results indicate a continued increase in pleural empyema in patients with AP, even in regions with developed health systems (70,71).

The development of the SARS-CoV-2 pandemic and the emergence of a new variant of COVID-19 pneumonia did not change the strategy for solving the problem of lung tissue inflammation. The causative agent of the process and its suppression continue to serve as the main goal for ongoing research and therapeutic efforts. The mechanisms of disease development are being studied mainly at the cellular and molecular level in the hope of finding ways to block the penetration of coronavirus into cells. However, the results of such searches can help mainly in the prodromal period. When clinical signs of the disease appear, treatment is limited to symptomatic, supportive and palliative measures. In this regard, A. H. Ottaway and co-authors rightly note that modern respiratory care revolves around auxiliary measures (16).

Meanwhile, new facts are emerging that only confirm the axiom that damage to the same structures is accompanied by a standard mechanism of functional disorders, and the pathogenetic mechanisms of viral pneumonia have the same basis as bacterial forms. For example, the use of tomography in patients with COVID-19 pneumonia to determine the volume of blood in the lungs allowed us to establish a decrease in this indicator in small vessels with a diameter of no more than 2 mm (93). The authors suggest that this fact is caused by spasm and thrombosis of small vessels as a result of their viral damage. Generalized thrombosis of this localization can hardly be compatible with life, but the spasm of the pulmonary vessels fully corresponds to the already known and mentioned above discharge reflex.

Such findings are considered as the result of viral damage without attempts to link the detected deviations with biological patterns and compensatory reactions of the body. The severity of the condition of patients with COVID-19 pneumonia is still explained by sepsis and septic shock without any evidence that circulatory disorders in these situations are really septic in nature and have no other causes (131-134). Previous interpretations of the basics of the problem retain the previous recommendations: mandatory intravenous infusions for such patients, and in case of insufficient effect - the use of vasopressors.

In conclusion, it is necessary to emphasize once again that the functional characteristics of blood circulation in the vessels of the small circulatory circle are the complete opposite of systemic blood flow, and the maintenance of the necessary vital proportions between the two circuits is carried out autonomously. In this regard, the pathogenesis of the consequences in the event of a violation of the circulation of pulmonary blood flow in AP will have a completely different character than the mechanisms of critical situations arising from inflammatory processes of other localization. Carrying out intravenous infusions with a substitutive or supportive purpose will have a completely different effect in AP, unlike other nosologies.

Thus, modern therapeutic efforts aimed at correcting systemic circulatory disorders in patients with AP are the result of an incorrect interpretation of their causes and mechanisms. The long-term "fascination" with antibiotic therapy in patients with AP has left a deep didactic trace with the oblivion of many biological laws, and the first step to solving the problem under discussion should be, first of all, bringing the concept of the disease in line with the basics of medical science.

CHAPTER 3

ADDITIONAL STUDIES OF THE MECHANISMS OF DEVELOPMENT AND COURSE OF ACUTE PNEUMONIA

3.1. Experimental studies

3.1.1. Why are experimental studies necessary?

The leading role of pathogens, their properties and influence on the structures and functions of the body have been the main areas of research in the study of the problem of AP for many years. The narrowness of this approach lies in the fact that an acute inflammatory process in the lungs is an example of conflicts that constantly arise in nature. Such clashes always involve at least two parties involved in the confrontation, and each of them contributes to this process. The development of AP marks a violation of parity between the microflora and the organism in which the latter is an active participant.

To date, many observations and facts have already been accumulated, indicating an infinite number of variants of the development of inflammatory processes in the conditions of a single monoinfection. Research in such situations usually focuses on the microbiological characteristics of the disease, but a number of cardinal questions about the body of patients still remain unanswered. Why are some patients with an identical assessment of their initial state of the body immune to the disease, while others literally burn out in a short time? What initial parameters can serve as a reliable prognostic test to determine the degree of aggressiveness of inflammation if this process suddenly occurs?

The list of such questions is grouped around the collision that occurs in certain situations between microflora and macroorganism. The necessary presence of certain conditions for the occurrence of AP is not a reservation, since the presence of even the most virulent strains in the body does not necessarily mean the development of an inflammatory process (72,74). In this regard, the claims that AP begins with the banal penetration of pathogenic microorganisms into the lung tissue should cause great doubts. However, this version of the development of bacterial forms of the disease remains working to this day and continues to be replicated in the literature.

WHO materials, which usually contain generalizing expert opinions, note that bacteria and viruses enter the lungs of patients with AP when inhaled (73). But, then a question immediately arises to the authors of these materials regarding the epidemiology of the disease, which is not provided for in this document in any way. Isolation of patients with lung damage and other precautions became recommended and even necessary only with the development of the SARS-CoV-2 pandemic and the emergence of a large contingent with COVID-19 pneumonia.

In addition, the question arises again, which has been raised more than once above, about why, with such an aggressive coronavirus, not everyone is susceptible to the disease, and 20% of infected people do not have any clinical manifestations at all (17-20). In such situations, when it is impossible to find the necessary answer in clinical conditions, research should be brought to the experimental level. Experiments cannot reproduce the environment around us absolutely accurately, but they allow us to recreate similar conditions and understand the main causes of the phenomenon being studied. In this context, it is necessary to present the information that was obtained by the author during the experimental reproduction of the model of acute bacterial inflammation of the lung tissue (135).

3.1.2. Reproduction of a model of acute bacterial inflammation in the lungs

The experiments were carried out in the experimental laboratory of the Novokuznetsk State Institute of Postgraduate Training of Doctors (Novokuznetsk, USSR) in the eighties of the last century. Unlike the State and institute where experimental studies were conducted and which have now ceased to exist in the previous version, the results of this work can provide useful information for assessing and understanding current events. Despite the considerable period of time that has passed since the completion of these studies, the author could not find such works in the world literature and is convinced that the information received has not lost its relevance, and if necessary, this search can be repeated and supplemented with new forms of tests.

The study was initiated due to a discrepancy between general views on the leading role of microbial aggression in the occurrence and development of AP and real facts with direct observation of the concentration of the most severe patients. In this regard, experimental research plans were initially focused on infecting lung tissue with microflora in order to assess the very fact of bacterial penetration into an area that was previously considered sterile. Only in recent years have the results of studies appeared that show the probability of the presence of an entire microbiological community in the bronchial tree of healthy people, including *streptococcus pneumoniae* (136).

The experiments were carried out on 44 rabbits weighing 3-4 kg. In total, 4 series of tests were conducted. The initial experimental manipulation in all animals was endobronchial instillation of various mixtures. These manipulations were performed under sterile conditions under intravenous sedation with thiopental. Piercing the trachea on the anterior surface of the neck, a polyvinyl chloride catheter with a diameter of 0.6 mm was inserted through the needle. The distal end of the catheter was moved to the required depth in the direction of small bronchial branches in one of the lungs. After infusion of the mixture, the catheter was immediately removed. The liquid mixture for infusions in each series of experiments differed in volume and proportions. The following materials were used as ingredients for the preparation of the primary mixture:

1. One billion of microbial bodies of one-day culture Staphylococcus epidermidis in 1 ml saline;
2. One billion of microbial bodies of one-day culture Escherichia coli in 1 ml saline;
3. Sterile sunflower oil;
4. Normal horse serum was added starting from 2nd series of experiments.

The choice of cultures of the above-mentioned microorganisms for experiments was made intentionally, since these bacteria were usually not included in the list of pathogens of AP. Thus, the experiment pursued the following goals:

- check the probability of developing AP with the participation of microorganisms that are not considered pathogens of the disease, and their detection is considered an accidental finding or the result of contamination and errors during bacteriological studies;
- definition of the role of other factors in the occurrence of non-specific inflammation of the lungs.

Autopsies of all experimental animals were performed after their death or euthanasia. The lungs of the animals were subjected to macro-and microscopic examination. Statistical evaluation of the results of the study was carried out according to successive test plans, as well as the method of controlling the average variance in pairs (137). These statistical methods allowed to limit the amount of experiments to obtain reliable results.

In the **first experimental series** (11 animals), the lung tissue was infected with an additional violation of bronchial patency. The liquid mixture contained 1 ml of Staphylococcus epidermidis culture, 0.5 ml of Escherichia coli culture and 1 ml of sterile sunflower oil; it was instilled through a catheter into the bronchial tree. On the second and third days of the experiment, seven animals were given slow jet intravenous infusions of reomacrodex (30 CC / kg body weight). All the animals were euthanized on the fourth day.

Partial atelectasis of the lung tissue was detected in all animals of this experimental series. No signs of acute inflammation were found in the lung tissue. Differences in the state of the lung tissue in animals receiving intravenous infusion were also not found. Thus, a simple infection of the lung tissue in the experiment, even under conditions of additional bronchial obstruction, was not accompanied by the development of acute inflammation.

The experiment conditions were changed in the **2nd series** (10 animals). All rabbits were given 5 ml of normal equine serum subcutaneously 7 days before endobronchial procedures. Endobronchial instillations included 1 ml of the same serum, followed by the ingredients as in the first series of experiments (1 ml of Staphylococcus epidermidis culture, 0.5 ml of Escherichia coli culture and 1 ml of sterile sunflower oil). 2 rabbits died within hours of the procedure with the clinic of severe pulmonary edema. Intravenous infusions (the same as in series 1) were performed on 6 animals on the 2nd and 4th days of the experiment. Euthanasia of animals that remained alive was performed on the 5th day.

Examination of the lungs revealed in all cases a diffuse vascular reaction corresponding to the picture of a "shock lung". No inflammatory changes characteristic of AP were detected. The results of the 2nd series of experiments showed that the introduction of a massive dose of a substance that was previously used to sensitize the body causes a rapid and severe allergic reaction from the pulmonary vessels. The infectious factor did not have a specific effect on the pathological picture.

Based on the results of the previous series, additional changes were made to the experience conditions. All 8 animals of the **3rd series** also received subcutaneous injections of 5 ml of horse serum a week before the manipulation. The main part of the experiment involved endobronchial administration of a smaller dose (0.2 ml) of horse serum and 0.5 ml of sunflower oil. Then 1 ml of Escherichia coli culture was administered intravenously.

In this series of experiments, a model of acute inflammation in the lung tissue was obtained, but this form of inflammation, from our point of view, had signs of hematogenic (septic) damage. So, shortly after the endobronchial procedure and intravenous infection, 3 animals died. Intravenous infusion was performed in 4 animals on the 2nd and 3rd days of the experiment. 3 animals of the last group died immediately after the end of the infusion. Euthanasia of 2 surviving animals was performed on the 4th day. Lung research revealed disseminated bilateral pneumonia in all animals in this series. The revealed pathoanatomic findings fully corresponded to the picture of septic pneumonia.

The main goal of the experimental work-to obtain a model of bronchogenic lung inflammation-was achieved only in the last, **4th series**. Experiments in this series were conducted on 15 animals. The main part of the experiment in all animals was the same. All rabbits were given 5 ml of normal equine serum subcutaneously seven days before the main part of the experiment. Then, using the method described above, the mixture was instilled endobronchially. The results of the previous two series with a pronounced vascular reaction forced us to significantly reduce the dose of serum for administration to the bronchi. This minuscule volume (0.05 ml) was mixed with 1 ml of Staphylococcus epidermidis culture and 1 ml of sunflower oil before administration.

In the future, the animals were divided into 2 groups. Seven animals (**series 4A**) did not receive additional manipulations. The remaining 8 animals (**series 4B**) received intravenous infusions. These infusions were performed 3-4 hours after endobronchial administration and then repeated once a day. In six animals from the last group, a dye (2 ml of methylene blue) was added to the solution for intravenous infusions. All animals were euthanized on the fourth day after endobronchial instillations.

The Staphylococcus epidermis was deliberately chosen as a microbial factor. This microbe does not belong to the category of particularly aggressive forms. This choice reduces the probability of the influence of aggressive qualities of the pathogen on the picture of the process and allows us to assess the role of other factors in the etiology of the disease. Thus, a typical macroscopic picture of macrofocal pneumonia was found in all 7 animals of the 4A series. The term "macrofocal" means that acute inflammation covers most of one of the lobes of the lung. Thin films of fibrin on the visceral pleura were found in 3 cases. Histological examination of lung preparations confirmed the presence of acute inflammation. In addition, in 1 case, small areas of necrosis were found in the area of inflammation.

The results obtained in Series 4A draw attention to the following important facts. Firstly, one of the most important causes of the inflammatory reaction was the contact of the lung tissue with a certain material after a preliminary "acquaintance" with it of the whole organism. Such contact caused a local tissue reaction, and the presence of microflora increased the inflammatory component of the process. Secondly, despite the strict repetition of the experimental conditions in each animal, the final results differed in the intensity of inflammatory changes and reflected the individual reaction of the body in each case. Finally, extensive inflammatory changes, including foci of necrosis, were obtained with the participation of microflora, which is usually not considered as the causative agent of the process in AP.

Of course, the results of experimental studies can not be fully considered as a mirror image of the conditions and situations observed in clinical practice. However, experimental medicine was created and continues to function in order to bring the experimental conditions as close as possible to the reproduction of natural phenomena in practical use, which are not fully understood and can not be tested at the patient 's bedside. Therefore, the results of such studies allow us to at least indirectly assess the significance of various factors in the Genesis of pathological processes.

As the descriptions of individual series of experiments show, the results depended on the selected conditions. One of the most important moments of the conducted research, in the end, was the allergization of the body of experimental animals. It was the effect of preliminary sensitization and repeated contact with the lung tissue that played a major role in the development of its acute lesion. At the same time, the final results depended on the repeated dose of the allergen, as well as on the ways of penetration of bacteria into the lungs.

Analysis of the results showed that the most realistic scenario for the occurrence of bronchogenic inflammatory process in lung tissue is the following brief interpretation. The basis for the occurrence of this pathology appears with an increase in the sensitivity of the body to certain substances, and the potential danger of developing AP increases, especially when the allergen is able to easily penetrate the lungs with inhaled air. The contact of such materials (antigens) with the structures of the lungs violates the protective mechanisms of the latter and causes a tissue reaction, the components and links of which are similar to the process of inflammation, in this regard, local allergic reactions are not accidentally designated by the term "allergic inflammation" (90,138). The presence or additional ingress of bacteria into this zone stimulates the further course of the process.

The importance of immune reactions in the development of AP is unlikely to be denied by anyone today. The range of manifestation of this reaction depends on the individual potential, and lifelong changes of the latter occur under the influence of an allergic component. In turn, the predisposition to allergic reactions increases with an increase in the load on the body's immune system as a result of increased contact with certain substances. In particular, the peculiarity of the development of AP with a particularly severe course was observed by us in the course of this work, and one of the reasons for this phenomenon was the significant pollution of the air basin by industrial emissions. This fact was confirmed by comparing the number of patients and variants of AP development depending on the place of residence and the concentration of impurities in the air of different zones (135).

The influence of various factors on the formation of the body's reaction has various variants, which depend on the initial state of the body's immune forces. We did not set ourselves the task of establishing and comparing the initial state of immunity in experimental animals. However, as noted above, despite the strict observance of the experimental conditions, the results in each series had a noticeable difference between them. The only exception was the first series of experiments, in which no preliminary sensitization was carried out and no reactions of the body to manipulation were noted.

3.1.3. The effect of infusion therapy on the dynamics of experimental pneumonia

After achieving the possibility of stable obtaining a model of acute bronchogenic inflammation in the lung, a final series of experiments (4B) was initiated, in which the task was to clarify the role and significance of intravenous infusions in the dynamics of the inflammatory process.

The conditions for obtaining the AP model were described in detail above in a series of experiments 4A. In the next series 4B, these experimental conditions were supplemented with intravenous infusions of solutions. 8 animals of this series received intravenous jet slow infusions of rheomacrodex and 0.9% sodium chloride (in equal proportions with a total volume of 30 ml / kg of body weight) 3-4 hours after endobronchial procedures. Then these infusions were repeated once a day. Six animals from this group received solutions with the addition of a dye (2 ml of methylene blue). There was no premature death of animals in this series of experiments. All animals were euthanized on the fourth day after endobronchial instillations.

The results obtained in this series of experiments were very interesting and revealing. The development of AP with the presence of pleural changes was observed in all animals. Small foci of destruction in inflamed lung tissue were found in 6 animals. In 2 autopsy observations, a spontaneous breakthrough of foci of destruction into the pleural cavity with the development of pyopneumothorax was diagnosed. The addition of a dye to the solution was borrowed from the experiments of V. Menkin, who at one time used this technique to determine the permeability factor (139). The dye used in infusion solutions stained the lung tissue along the periphery of the inflammatory zone, creating a marking of the spread of the inflammatory process around the initial infiltration (Fig. 6).

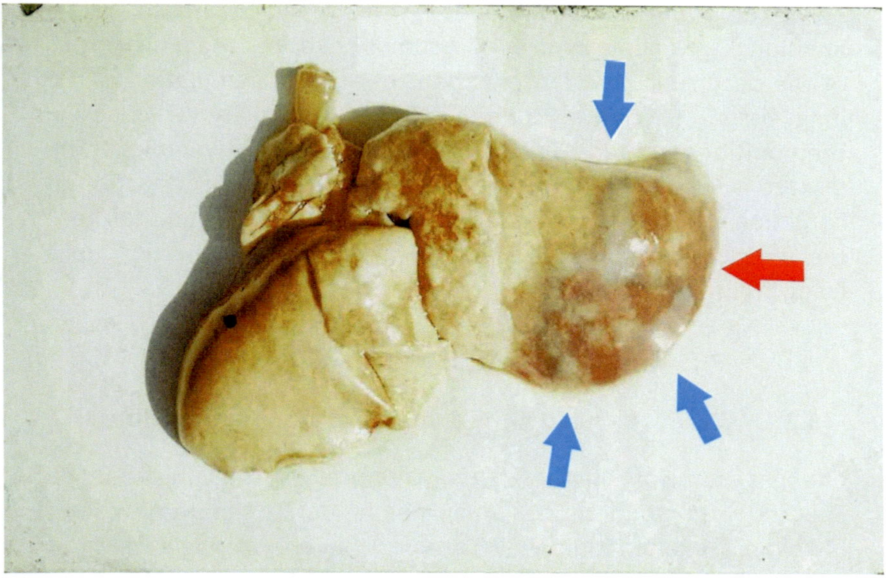

Figure 6. Lung macropreparation, experiment, series 4b. A massive focus of inflammation of the lung tissue (red arrow), surrounded by additional areas of infiltration with a blue tint (blue arrows).

According to the results of this series of experiments, an author's certificate was obtained for the invention of a model of parapneumonic pleurisy (140). The combination of the results of clinical observations and data from the last series of experiments made it possible to speak with more confidence about the negative effect of intravenous infusions on the dynamics of AP and to regard this factor as iatrogenic. In the initial period of AP, when there is an active process of edema and tissue infiltration, intravenous fluid administration can have a particularly strong stimulating effect on the dynamics of inflammation in the lungs. Regardless of the place of infusion, intravenously administered solutions are directed directly to the area of lung damage (Fig. 3). Even a minimal increase in returning blood to the area of increasing edema and tissue infiltration can give an additional incentive to these processes.

Thus, the results of experimental studies allowed us to obtain additional arguments in favor of assumptions about the mechanisms of the occurrence and development of acute inflammation in the lung tissue. In clinical conditions, the probability of checking premonitions and guesses about the features of the dynamics of the disease is very complex and problematic. Artificial reproduction of conditions close to those observed in the clinic allows you to check the effect of certain biological phenomena in the conditions of a living organism.

3.2. X-ray anatomical studies of the lungs.

3.2.1. Why do we need X-ray anatomical studies of the lungs?

Changes occurring in the tissue structures of the lungs can be checked and studied in detail mainly during anatomical and histological examination, which are possible only during autopsy or in rare cases as a result of surgical interventions. However, even with such a fairly accurate version of the study, the proportions between the individual structures of organs that change during the pathological transformation of tissues are almost impossible to track and establish. The study of these patterns is important information for understanding not so much the anatomical as the functional consequences of the inflammatory process, since the axiom of the inseparable connection of morphological and functional characteristics remains one of the fundamental in the living biological world.

In order to fill in the gaps in obtaining information about new anatomical relationships between the structures of lung tissue in conditions of acute inflammation, X-ray anatomical studies were conducted. X-ray anatomical studies were carried out on 56 whole anatomical lung preparations that were taken for this study during the autopsy of children who died from AP. In 9 cases, the bronchi were contrasted. A separate contrast of pulmonary vessels (arteries or veins) was performed on 47 samples, followed by X-ray examination. All these studies were conducted as follows.

The procedure was performed immediately after opening and extracting the sample, which was not subjected to any additional influences. A catheter intended for medical purposes was inserted into the initial part of the main bronchus or the corresponding vessel and strictly fixed in this position with an external silk ligature. The catheter had a cannula at the distal end through which a liquid contrast agent was injected with a syringe. For contrast studies, drugs that are usually used in the clinic for diagnostic purposes by intravenous administration were used. Contrast was injected with light pressure on the plunger of the syringe until the first signs of resistance appeared. The X-ray was taken immediately after discontinuation of contrast agent administration.

3.2.2. X-ray anatomy of the bronchial tree in acute pneumonia

Violation of bronchial patency and its restoration occupies an important place in the pathogenesis of AP, since the loss of ventilation and airiness of the lung tissue, as well as their restoration, are directly related to the condition of the corresponding areas of the bronchial tree. The frequent presence of easily expressed signs of respiratory syndrome in the form of a cough, sometimes barely noticeable, before the onset of pneumonia indicates the presence of tracheoendobronchitis. Such endobronchial inflammation without significant clinical manifestations does not attract much attention, but it should be borne in mind that such a syndrome can cause ventilation disorders and often precedes inflammation of the lung tissue. In addition, it should be borne in mind that this fact (?) is usually established on the basis of a patient's survey. Many of them do not pay serious attention to these "insignificant" signs that remain behind the scenes of events.

The presence of inflammatory processes in the lower respiratory tract, even with subtle symptoms, in any case suggests at least three main factors, the appearance of which narrows the lumen of the bronchi. Inflammation of the bronchial mucosa is accompanied by its swelling and thickening. The production of bronchial secretions increases, which is not immediately removed from the bronchial lumen. In the small branches of the bronchial tree, which do not have such a powerful cough reflex as the larynx and trachea, the secret can linger for a considerable time. In response to inflammation, the tone of the bronchial muscles increases, the relative proportion of which in the anatomical structure and their role in bronchospasm increase as the diameter of the bronchi decreases.

In connection with the last remarks, it should be noted that a serious disadvantage of the bronchial obstruction method in the experiments described above is a purely physical version of reproducing such an obstacle without an inflammatory component. If it were possible to create a preliminary picture of a mild respiratory syndrome in the experiment, and then transfer the process to the stage of inflammation of the lung tissue, then the conditions of such testing would, from my point of view, be the closest to real observations. This digression refers primarily to the first series of experiments.

It should be added to the above that the occurrence and development of the inflammatory process in the lung tissue is accompanied not only by the appearance and accumulation of inflammatory exudate in the alveoli, but also by inflammatory infiltration and edema of the lung tissue itself. The latter circumstance is another factor that can block small bronchial branches due to their external compression by the inflammatory expansion of surrounding tissues.

The maximum possible information about the state of the bronchial tree in the focus of inflammation is necessary in order to have an idea of the degree and depth of its disorders. This information makes it possible to clarify possible ways to restore bronchial patency, without which it is unthinkable to return ventilation and normal respiratory functions to those areas of lung tissue that were in the area of inflammation.

A contrast study of the bronchial tree, which was carried out on 9 lung preparations in children who died from AP, in all cases revealed a complete blockage of the bronchi in the area of inflammation (Fig. 7).

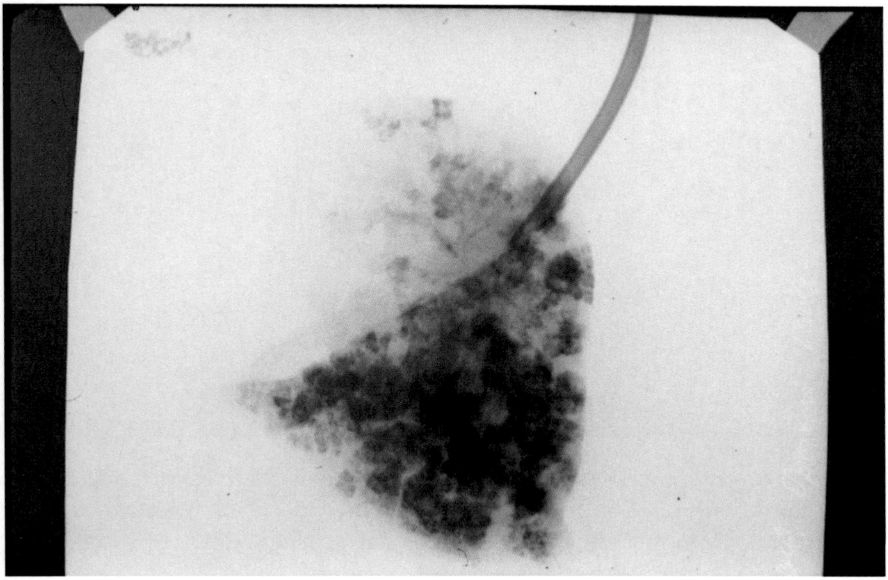

Figure 7. Bronchogram of the left lung preparation with total inflammation of the upper lobe. The contrast agent filled most of the lower lobe to the alveolar level, but almost did not penetrate the bronchi of the upper lobe.

The presented results coincided with the lifetime contrast of the tracheobronchial tree, which was performed during the control of microtracheostomy after its imposition. The introduction of contrast made it possible to determine the localization of the inner end of the catheter. MTS was used as one of the methods of intensive restoration of bronchial patency, and the greatest effect of its action was achieved when a catheter was installed in the tracheal bifurcation area, which contributed to the most active cough. A total of 44 such studies were conducted. Contrasting of the bronchial tree in these patients also revealed blocking of branches in the area of inflammation (Fig. 8).

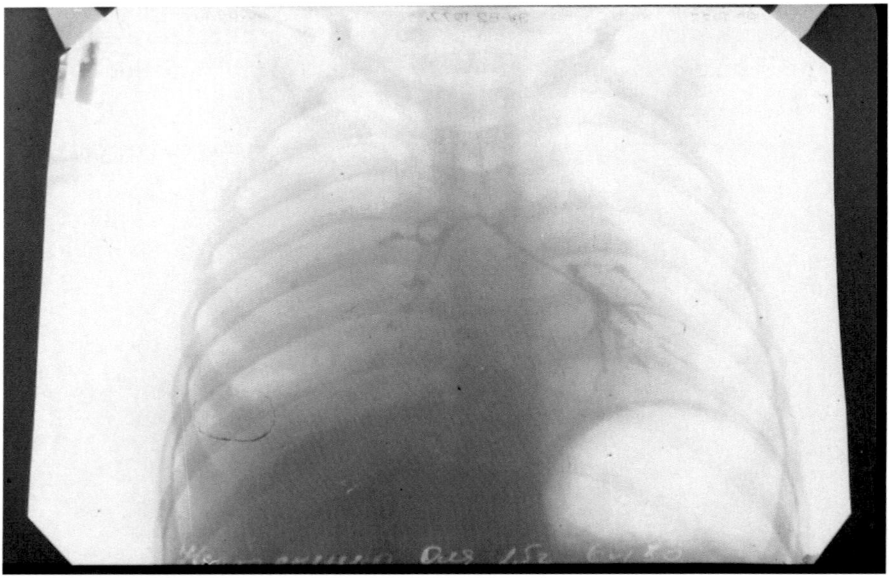

Figure 8. Patient with AP in the lower lobe of the right lung. Introduction of contrast through microtracheostomy. The bronchi of the right lung contrast only in the initial sections. The contrast agent did not penetrate into the area of inflammation.

Thus, the results of various contrast studies of bronchial patency in AP allow us to note that the lumen of the bronchial tree in the area of inflammation is constantly blocked as a result of the influence of various factors. This fact is important information for choosing medical care options for such patients.

3.2.3. Angioarchitectonics of acute pneumonia

The onset of an acute inflammatory reaction in the lung tissue means the consistent development of pathological restructuring of the vascular bed and corresponding changes in blood flow in the affected area. This transformation has been studied in detail in inflammation as a whole (90), and its classical manifestation in the lungs is most clearly represented when the entire lobe is affected (141,142). Changes in the diameter of the vessels, the proportions between the arterial and venous sectors and the subsequent slowing of blood flow occur under conditions of a sharp increase in the permeability of the vascular wall and diffusion of the internal contents of the vessels into the surrounding tissues.

Initially, the inflammatory reaction is manifested by the emerging arterial hyperemia with increased blood flow to the area of inflammation and increased vascular permeability. These processes lead to edema and inflammatory infiltration of surrounding tissues with an increase in their volume. Such changes are accompanied by an increase in the external pressure of the surrounding tissues on the blood vessels. The result of such external pressure is first manifested in a more flexible vascular segment with lower blood pressure. Therefore, at the first stages of the development of the inflammatory process, the primary compression of the venous sections of the vascular bed occurs while maintaining increased blood flow through the arteries.

As a result of the described changes in blood flow in the area of acute inflammation, at a certain stage of their development, an additional mechanism occurs that stimulates edema and infiltration of tissues in the affected area. This mechanism, which supports the flow of blood to the focus of inflammation and prevents its outflow, creates the conditions of the so-called "vascular trap". We found the basis for the action of such a mechanism in the affected area of AP and confirmed this with additional studies of lung drugs that were taken from patients who died from AP with varying degrees of pathological changes in the lung tissue. This mechanism of transformation in the area of inflammation can operate within the preserved blood flow. Stopping the blood flow marks the beginning of irreversible damage to tissue structures and is further defined as foci of destruction.

Variations of the revealed changes in the architectonics of the vascular bed are shown in the illustrations (Fig. 9-11).

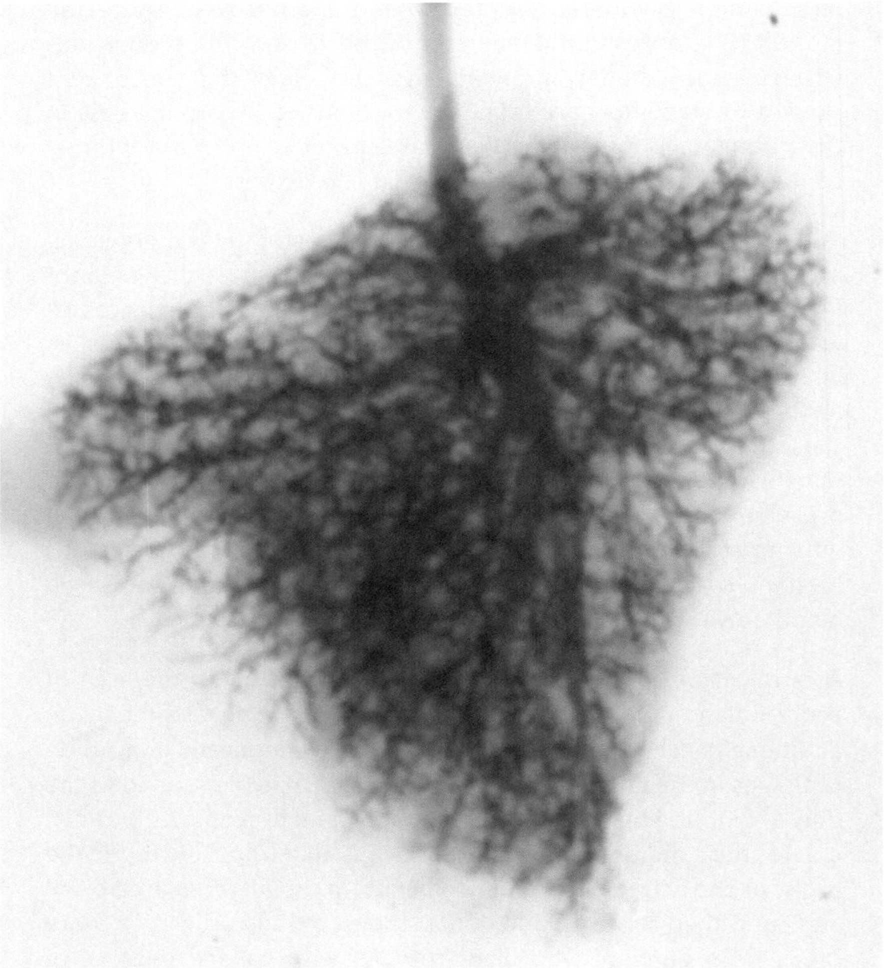

Figure 9. Arteriogram of a lung preparation with total inflammation of the lower lobe (histological examination revealed no signs of necrosis). The contrast is evenly distributed across the arteries of all parts of the lung.

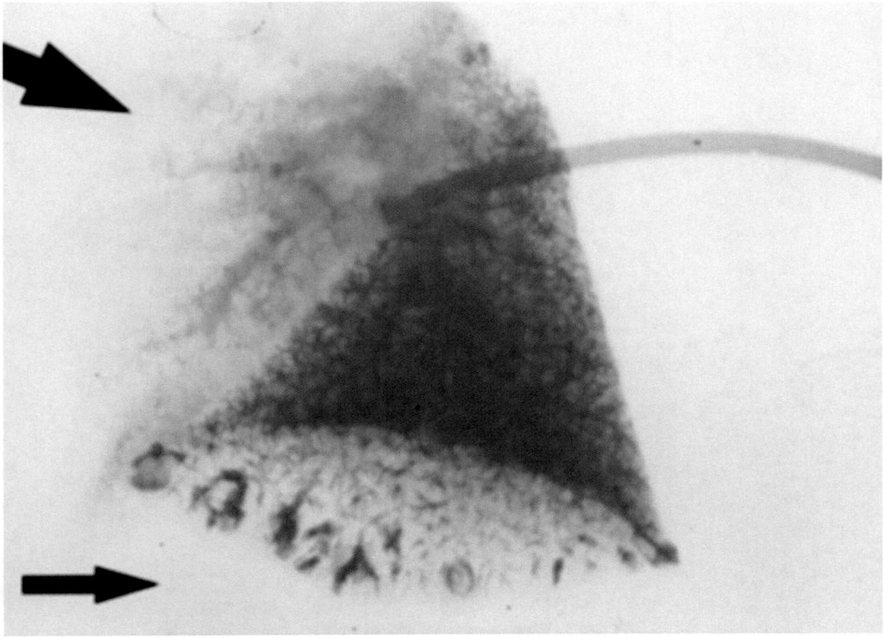

Figure 10. Contrasting the veins of the lung preparation with a massive focus of inflammation in the upper lobe (subsequent histology revealed no signs of necrosis in the area of inflammation). There is no penetration of contrast agent into the veins of the upper lobe of the lung (large arrow). The venous network of the lower lobe is well contrasted, and relatively large semicircular vascular formations are visible in its basal sections (small arrow).

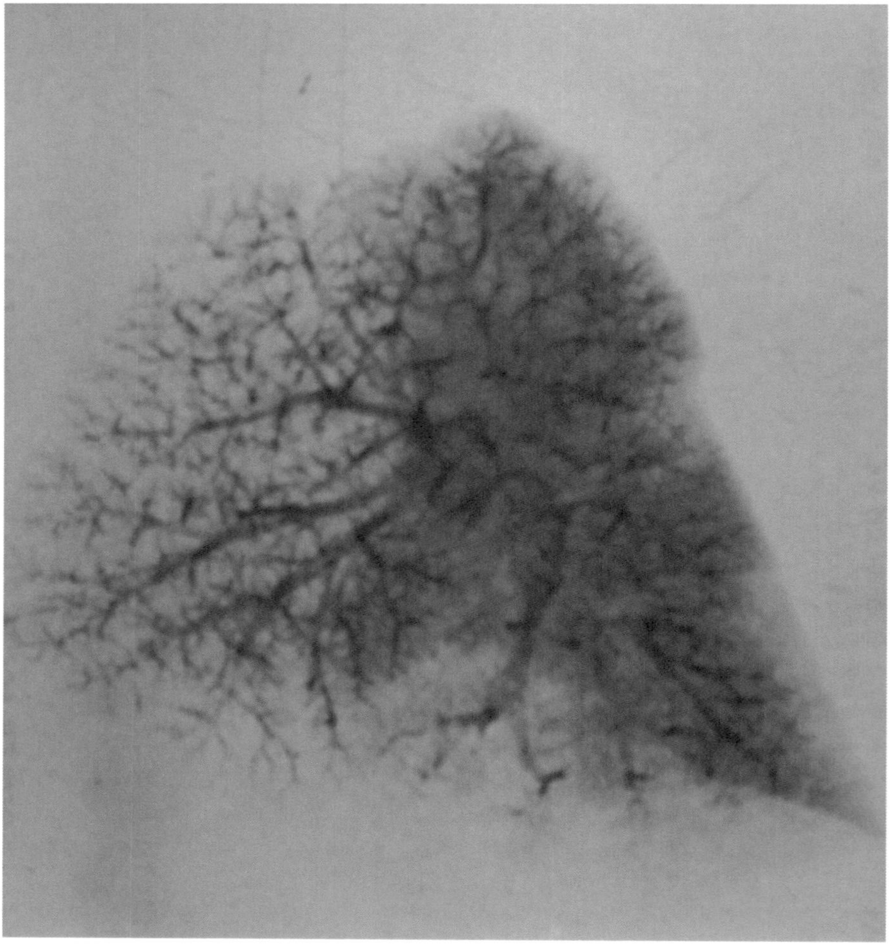

Figure 11. Arteriogram of the lung preparation with foci of necrosis in the peripheral parts of the lower lobe. The contrast did not fill the peripheral network of blood vessels in some parts of the lower lobe.

Thus, a contrast study of the vessels of the small circulatory circle at various stages of inflammatory changes in the lung showed the following. As a result of the inflammatory transformation of tissues, a peculiar mechanism of "vascular trap" arises, which contributes to the further development of edema and infiltration of tissues in case of preservation of blood flow to this zone. Even a slight increase in the volume of flowing blood can accelerate the current processes with the cessation of blood flow in inflamed tissues and their necrosis. Such a mechanism develops in parallel with the degree of pathological transformation of tissues in the area of inflammation, and the revealed radiological data depend more on the intensity of the development of the process than on the variant of its etiology.

CHAPTER 4

DISCUSSION OF THE DOCTRINE OF ACUTE PNEUMONIA

4.1. Why is it necessary to reconsider the ideology of acute pneumonia?

Our understanding of the nature of AP, the causes and mechanisms of its development determines the further direction of therapeutic efforts and the final results. When the results of treatment do not meet the expected ones, it is considered as an incorrect choice of drugs, their dosages or a consequence of other tactical omissions. If the reasons for the insufficient effectiveness of AP treatment were precisely defects in the choice of tactics or pharmaceuticals, then correcting such inconsistencies would make it possible to quickly close this topic. However, dissatisfaction with the treatment of this disease continues to grow for many years, and there are no reasoned explanations for this phenomenon. The main goal of efforts is still the causative agent of the process, which must be identified and suppressed.

For several decades, the effectiveness of treatment of patients with AP has been slowly but steadily declining, and attempts to correct this negative trend by constantly updating the range of antimicrobials as the main therapeutic agent have not significantly affected the results. The concern of specialists all over the world about the negative trend of the course of this disease and the growth of its complicated forms did not go beyond the statement of facts, and the lack of explanations for the observed phenomena remained without a radical search for answers and continued to revolve around the etiotropic principles of medical care (59,65,66,143-145).

In this regard, it is necessary to understand that therapeutic principles do not arise from a vacuum. They are formed on the basis of our ideas about the nature and features of a particular disease. For example, if one drug therapy is clearly not enough for patients with skeletal fractures, then seeing the need for surgical intervention in every patient with abdominal pain is clearly too much, isn't it? Conceptual ideas about the nature of each disease are actually a strategy for solving its problem.

During many years of focusing on the effect of antibacterial therapy, the strategy for solving the problem of AP has been reduced to the concept of a single task, in which the whole essence of the solution is determined by the etiology of the disease. But the concept of etiology has a much broader meaning, therefore, to be more precise, a purely antibacterial approach was formed to take the necessary measures. However, as reality shows, the development of the SARS-CoV-2 pandemic and the breaking of established therapeutic stereotypes have exposed chaotic ideas about ways out of the current situation. It turns out that the very concept of "strategy", in relation to the problem of AP, can have a variety of options and interpretations.

Currently, many articles are being published on the topic of acute inflammation of the lung tissue, in which the question of changing strategic directions in this problem is raised and specific proposals are made. However, a detailed acquaintance with the proposed plans of strategic solutions shows that in such messages the strategy of the problem is not discussed at all, but we are talking about tactical steps, organizational measures or simply switching attention to certain drugs.

In the current coronavirus pandemic, the most acute problem is the care of patients with COVID-19 pneumonia, which turned out to be possible only at the level of auxiliary and supportive techniques. In this regard, the increase in the number of articles on this topic containing various versions of the new strategy looks quite logical.

Unfortunately, from my point of view, among the many proposals, there was not one that would be a truly strategic solution, and the concept of the disease is not even questioned, continuing to consider the causative agent of the process as the main and, in fact, the only cause.

For example, it is hardly possible to find opponents of effective prevention of the disease, since it is always more difficult to treat the process that has already arisen and it is not always possible to achieve the full effect. But declaring prevention of coronavirus pneumonia the best strategy, while patients with this pathology receive medical support instead of guaranteed treatment, does not look at all like a targeted offer (38). Or a strategic declaration on the creation of obstacles to the penetration of viruses into cells (43,44)? This proposal is also an option for preventing the disease, rather than treating those who are already ill. Moreover, there are no ways to implement such an idea yet, and the authors have not developed it either.

Or, for example, can maintaining a certain level of vitamin D in the body be considered as a new strategy to combat coronavirus disease? But in the end, this sentence is clothed in this form (41). Timely intubation of patients and their connection to artificial lung ventilation, as well as, if necessary, the use of extracorporeal membrane oxygenation of blood are also presented as a new strategic solution (39).

However, the largest number of strategic proposals presenting options for a global solution to the pandemic crisis due to the sharp increase in the number of patients with COVID-19 pneumonia is associated with the problem of meeting the needs for providing artificial ventilation devices (146-148) and improving care for the insufficiency of other systems (42). In this regard, a logical question arises: if a person has lost the respiratory function of the lungs as a result of a disease and a technique is used to save him, which replaces this loss, is such a step a strategic solution to the problem?

Or is it still substitution and maintenance therapy? I am deeply convinced that in this case the last option is being discussed, which is not even radical in nature.

In order to understand the essence of such misconceptions, we can give a similar example with the loss of another function of the body. For example, for some reason, the function of the lower extremities is temporarily lost and auxiliary means are used for the necessary movement of the patient. However, such replacement assistance can hardly be considered a strategic solution to the reason why this problem arose, can it?

The fundamental difference between these two situations is that in the first case we are talking about a violation of a vital function, without the preservation of which a fatal outcome is inevitable. Nevertheless, maintaining the lost function at the required level, artificial ventilation does not affect the cause that caused it, and, of course, does not eliminate it. Moreover, it has already been established that intubation and subsequent artificial ventilation of the lungs are accompanied by a significantly higher mortality rate (19,209), therefore, strengthening this auxiliary care is not of strategic importance. At the same time, attention should be paid to such a sign as the absence of a direct relationship between the parameters of the source of respiratory failure and the degree of the latter.

It is believed that the main cause of respiratory dysfunction and gas exchange disorders in AP is the inflammatory process of the alveolar parts of the organ, which creates an obstacle to the diffusion of gases. However, on the other hand, it is known that one patient can maintain relatively adequate breathing with 60% damage to lung tissue, and the other needs intubation and auxiliary ventilation with a noticeably smaller volume of inflammation. That is, the mechanisms of the development of the pathological process in the lung are more complex than they usually seem.

In addition to a number of existing but unexplained inconsistencies between the ideology of the AP and the observed facts, the development of the SARS-CoV-2 pandemic has added new problems to them. Now patients with coronavirus pneumonia pose an epidemic danger to others, and antibiotics, without which many cannot imagine a reliable treatment, have lost their former importance without a decent antiviral replacement. At the same time, we continue to talk about one nosological form, which in recent decades has again changed its leader among its pathogens, while retaining all the signs characteristic of AP (118,149-151).

Today, the whole world is looking for the optimal solution in a pandemic, trying to get out of it with the least losses. Every practitioner is faced with an unresolved issue: "What can and should be done to effectively help patients with COVID-19 pneumonia?" Due to established traditions, everyone hopes for success in the development of antiviral drugs, continuing to ignore the already accumulated experience of antibiotic therapy, which has shown that with the aggressive development of the etiotropic treatment process, this is clearly not enough to achieve success. While everyone is waiting and hoping for a successful result of the search for etiotropic drugs, medical care is symptomatic and supportive, and its effectiveness everywhere, regardless of the level of local medicine, leaves much to be desired.

In recent years, the effectiveness of the treatment of bacterial forms of AP continued to decline slowly, but the dynamics of this process remained without a reasoned interpretation. The usual explanations for this phenomenon were the virulence of the microflora, the growth of its resistance, difficulties in determining the pathogens of AP and a decrease in the activity of antibiotics. That is, attention was still focused on the etiology of the disease and its etiotropic treatment. Against this background, the coronavirus invasion was perceived as a terrible catastrophe with grave consequences. This assessment is correct, but only with the caveat that this event did not affect the effectiveness of treatment of this group of patients.

For example, mortality among seriously ill patients with COVID-19 pneumonia remained at the same level that was recorded in recent years with bacterial forms of AP (21-29).

A number of recent events are unequivocal evidence of the fact that the view of the problem under discussion as the result of infection alone is too limited and does not reflect reality. Within the framework of the current SARS-CoV-2 pandemic, it has already become quite obvious that the entry of coronavirus into the body is very far from the concept of a mandatory disease. If with bacterial forms of AP there was a theoretical possibility to explain the different severity of the disease by the presence of different pathogens, today, in conditions of monoinfection, patients continue to differ significantly in their clinical symptoms. In this situation, the preservation of the previous worldview on AP, which has developed under the influence of the action of antibiotics, seems clearly short-sighted and erroneous.

In all areas of professional activity, the success of the tasks set depends on the accepted system of views, which is designated by the term "doctrine". The essence of this term and its content determine the worldview on a specific problem and the resulting guiding principle of the solution (152). In this context, the definition and content of the AP doctrine should be considered as the basis for solving the problem of this disease.

In the available modern descriptions of AP, regardless of the volume and form of publication, such a section as the doctrine of the disease, as a rule, does not appear at all. The basis of the system of views on this problem can be judged only by the accents in the presentation of the presented material. The main attention is usually paid to the causes of AP, which repeat the bacterial section of its etiology. Therefore, the most important information about the nature of AP is usually not the doctrine of the disease, but a list of its possible microbial pathogens with a description of their pathogenic qualities. The next important section of such descriptions is a list of the optimal choice of antibiotics depending on the suspected pathogens.

Discussion of the leading role of individual pathogens in the etiology of AP is not combined with the actual results of this type of diagnosis, since the vast majority of patients in this group remain without establishing the microbial causes of the disease (2,59,60). The etiology of AP is often determined using biomarkers and other indirect signs that reflect the presence of a microbe in the patient's body, but do not prove its participation in the inflammatory process. Even positive results of bacteriological studies from the affected area with purulent complications are of dubious value and reliability, since against the background of long-term antibacterial therapy, a change of microorganisms can occur by this period of the disease, and often their complete disappearance.

The human body is a complex self-regulating system. In the process of vital activity, deviations and autonomous regulation of various functions and their constants constantly occur. No one in everyday life is engaged in conscious (!) constant monitoring and regulation of blood pressure, gastrointestinal secretion and peristalsis, excretory activity of the kidneys, right? These processes occur autonomously due to existing mechanisms. Our professional knowledge in this field is quite extensive, but this knowledge is not always used properly.

Knowledge and evaluation of the most important compensatory and adaptive mechanisms that play a crucial role in various diseases is only an introductory part of the information. It is necessary to have a detailed understanding of the sequence of processes taking place, as well as the limits of permissible deviations when compensatory reactions retain their positive effect and when they acquire negative qualities that require external assistance and additional correction. The permissible limit of the observed shifts in the course of the disease is the so-called "norm in pathology", when obvious deviations in the body's constants reflect the peculiarity of compensatory shifts, thanks to which the body's ability to resist the disease is preserved. An attempt to correct and normalize such indicators and conditions can destroy the protective system and bring it out of balance.

Despite the undoubted fact that the danger of AP development is caused by a violation of vital functions of the body, the idea of the mechanisms of disease development today is focused on information about the cellular and molecular level of the processes taking place. This trend in the study of the problem is primarily due to the fact that the main cause of the disease is considered to be its causative agent. In this regard, an intensive search continues for the leading mechanisms of damage to cellular structures and ways to neutralize these causes.

Such an emphasis in the study of the problem leaves without proper interest the causes of integrative systemic disorders, as well as the interaction and interdependence of various body systems with each other during the disease. The current tendency to seek a solution to the problem at the microscopic level and to develop a drug treatment option for AP immediately loses its priority in case of deterioration of the patient's condition and the appearance of critical signs. In such situations, creative imagination gives way to already proven pragmatic efforts to maintain systemic violations. It was such actions that gave and continue to give hope to the most difficult patients.

The modern problem of medical care for patients with AP begins with the concept of disease. The prevailing worldview about the exclusively infectious nature of this problem ignores the results of many classical materials of medical science. Inflammation, which was and is the main distinguishing feature of AP as a nosological form, begins to be replaced by a judgment about infection with a specific pathogen, and the pathogenic qualities of the latter begin to be considered as the main causes of clinical symptoms.

Discussing the basics of septic complications, the experts came to the conclusion that the terms "inflammation" and "inflammatory reaction" are overly widely used in assessing the condition of the most severe patients with inflammatory processes and focused on the definitions of "sepsis" and "septic shock" (85,86). However, since the analysis of patients with AP is carried out on the basis of criteria common with other nosologies, the number of septic complications without their bacteriological confirmation among lung patients began to grow. At the same time, the role of the inflammatory process in pneumonia remains the same, and its typical signs in COVID-19 remain to the same extent as in bacterial forms (38,118,149,153).

The inevitable disorders of the vital activity of an inflamed organ cover all its inherent functions. Today, functional disorders in AP are assessed mainly from the point of view of the blockade of alveolar gas exchange. The important location and function of the lungs in the circulatory system do not affect the interpretation of the pathogenetic features of AP. When assessing this disease, this lung function and its change in conditions of acute inflammation remain without due attention.

Prejudice in the infectious nature of the disease and accumulated omissions in its features continue to be reproduced today with the help of educational programs, methodological recommendations and regulatory documents. These circumstances further deepen the essence of the problem, complicate its understanding and correction of existing omissions and contradictions on this issue. That is why the number one task at present is to bring the system of views on the problem of AP in line with the fundamental foundations of medical science. The results of this work will become a kind of guide for further targeted research on the way to the successful achievement of the main goal.

4.2. Substantiation of the main provisions of the doctrine of acute pneumonia

4.2.1. The essence of acute pneumonia: inflammation or infection?

AP is a classic example of acute inflammation of nonspecific etiology. The main and characteristic feature of the disease is the inflammatory process, which has evidence of its occurrence and development on the basis of clinical, laboratory, radiological and pathomorphological signs and criteria. The development of inflammation in the lung tissue is the essence of this disease. It is senseless and irrational to deny this fact, as well as to prove that the term "pneumonia" has nothing to do with the process of inflammation at all.

Despite the indisputability of the most important distinguishing feature of AP from many other pathologies, the importance of the inflammatory process in the development and course of this disease in recent years has been replaced by the dominant assumption of the leading role of the pathogen. Moreover, in some analytical materials on septic complications, experts note that the inflammatory process as a biological phenomenon is overrepresented in the assessment of clinical options and situations (85). At the same time, the concentration of attention and subsequent efforts on the pathogens of AP does not correspond to real circumstances and, most importantly, does not bring the desired results.

The first experience of using antibiotics gave the impression that the etiotropic effect is sufficient to achieve success in the treatment of AP. Over the subsequent period, there have been huge changes in the conditions for this type of therapy. The emergence and growth of the number of resistant strains stimulated the development and release of new generations of antibiotics, the action of which cannot repeat the initial effectiveness of their predecessors. In recent decades, the frequency of viral etiology diseases has begun to increase, in which antibiotics lose their therapeutic value. The intensification of all these circumstances for many years serves as a signal for a reassessment of the place of antibiotics in the treatment of AP. However, the paradox of today's situation is that, contrary to the facts, the importance of the pathogen in the development of the disease and its suppression for successful treatment are becoming more and more dominant concepts.

AP does not have its own specific type of pathogen. In the pre-antibiotic era, pneumococcus was considered the most frequent microorganism of the disease, but even at that time it was not the only bacterial factor of AP. After the introduction of antibiotics into practice, the list of predominant pathogens of AP began to change constantly. It is enough to recall the period of leadership of staphylococcus, which used to be a rare cause of inflammation of the lung tissue.

The presence of a wide bacterial spectrum in the etiology of AP and a noticeable decrease in the effectiveness of antimicrobial therapy led to titanic efforts to identify the causative agent of the disease as early as possible for targeted antibacterial therapy. As is known, this task has not been effectively solved, and after many years of attempts to use various options for bacterial diagnosis of AP, confessions began to appear that the results of such studies do not affect the success of treatment, and the use of antibiotics has been and remains empirical (6,15).

Unfortunately, even the AP diagnostics section did not avoid distorting its fundamental principles. In recent years, when suspected of AP, there has been a tendency, in the absence of radiological data, to interpret such results in favor of pneumonia, and such cases have begun to appear as radiologically negative (212-215). If we simplify the description of such information, it turns out that inflammation of the lung tissue exists without evidence of this fact. Logically, there should be a question about the legality and expediency of such a diagnosis. The answer to this question can be found in the same publications where such overdiagnosis of AP is explained by the need to ensure early use of antibiotics. That is, the mythical fear of the pathogen prevails over the rational understanding of the fact that the disease in question has not been proven.

The absence of a pathogen in the blood during septic complications of AP is not considered an obstacle to the diagnosis of sepsis or septic shock today, and these diagnoses, established only on the basis of analogies with other diseases, determine the nature of subsequent treatment. However, in the case of negative X-ray examinations with suspected inflammation of the lung tissue, it is still proposed to use computed tomography (216).

Thus, tomographic studies in 4% of layered sections excluded the presence of AP, but in 9% of cases allowed to establish a focus of inflammation that was not detected by conventional chest radiography. The latter circumstance may be associated not only with higher tomography capabilities. Usually, negative radiography results in patients with AP occur in situations where the study is limited to only one frontal projection. With this direction of the rays, the focus of inflammation in the basal parts of the lungs is often masked by the shadow of the diaphragm. Such causes of possible errors are well known and can be easily eliminated by performing lateral radiographs.

However, in this case we are not talking about the pros and cons of X-ray diagnostics, but about the so-called radionegative pneumonia. The discussion of the specifics of performing radiographs and additional tomography is rather academic in nature. In clinical practice, if AP is suspected and doubts remain about this diagnosis, as a rule, a decision is made in favor of prescribing antibiotics. At the same time, it's no secret that in outpatient settings, the appointment of antibiotics is not always preceded by an X-ray examination. The number of such outpatient patients whose diagnosis of AP remained unconfirmed, but they were treated with antibiotics, hardly anyone can accurately calculate.

The analysis of materials concerning X-ray negative pneumonia draws attention to an obvious paradox that belongs to this category of patients. On the one hand, X-ray examination of patients is used to detect inflammatory transformation of lung tissue. That is, the meaning of this study emphasizes the fundamental role of the focus of inflammation in the diagnosis of AP and the presence of inflammation of the lung tissue (regardless of its causative agent!) this is the main criterion of this disease.

On the other hand, the results of X-ray diagnostics do not affect the basic principle of medical care, which is aimed at suppressing the pathogen of the process. The empirical choice of antibiotics has been the basis of emergency care for patients with AP for many years, including monitoring of so-called X-ray negative cases of the disease, which emphasizes the therapeutic priority of fighting infection rather than eliminating the focus of inflammation.

In other words, the focus of inflammation in the lung tissue mainly serves today as an object for the diagnosis of AP, but its confirmation does not affect the solution of therapeutic tasks (except for the development of pulmonary or pleural complications). The main therapeutic efforts are directed against infection, although in many patients the pathogen remains unidentified, and not against the dynamics of the inflammatory process and its effect on the function of the affected organ. The reason for this distortion of priorities lies in the long-term reassessment of the therapeutic role of antibiotics and the didactic influence of this process.

If during the period of predominance of bacterial forms of inflammation, the desire to identify the causative agent of the process was still justified by the hope of the action of antibiotics, then with the development of the SARS-CoV-2 pandemic, the continuation of the previous traditions regarding the etiology of the disease and etiotropic treatment has no logical explanation. Now there is a large group of patients with COVID-19 pneumonia, in which antibiotics lose their purpose. Bacterial coinfection in these patients is detected in isolated cases, the reliability of its diagnostic methods remains in great doubt, but the vast majority of such viral pneumonia is treated with antibiotics (109-118). What is the logic of such actions? With such priorities, is it possible to object to the fact that the distortion of ideas about the nature of AP was formed under the influence of antibacterial therapy?

AP, which is based on an inflammatory process caused not only by various pathogens, but also by representatives of various microbiological classes, such as bacteria or viruses, retains the unity of its main features so much that their differential diagnosis based on etiology remains a very difficult and often unsolvable task (116-118, 217, 218). In this regard, to continue to support the thesis about the leading importance of the properties of the pathogen for the clinic of the disease looks at least groundless and short-sighted.

But the most surprising thing is that, if earlier differences in clinical manifestations and results of AP treatment were often explained by a probable difference in pathogens, now the same variety of variants is observed in the presence of a single pathogen. According to statistics, 80% of people infected with coronavirus endure this contact without medical assistance (a quarter of them without any external signs) and only 20% need hospitalization (17-20). Moreover, if there was hope for antibiotics before, at present an etiotropic treatment has not yet been found. In this situation, to adhere to the point of view that inhaling the pathogen into the lungs is enough for the development of pneumonia is too primitive and does not correspond to the real situation (73), and the presence of highly virulent strains in the body also does not necessarily mean the development of the disease (72,74).

AP pathogens are only one of the provoking factors of inflammation in the lung tissue, but not the main and only cause of the disease. Bacteria and viruses remain the leading pathogens of AP, and their list is quite extensive. The absence of one specific pathogen, the periodic and unpredictable change of leaders among them while maintaining the main signs and criteria of the disease reflects the nonspecific nature of the observed process.

Among the etiological factors of the so-called bronchogenic forms of AP, habitat and food quality play an important role, which affect the growth of allergic reactions (219-224). Increased sensitization of the population increases the risk of respiratory allergic diseases with repeated contacts of various allergens with the respiratory tract during breathing. This circumstance is reflected in an increase in the frequency of AP in the presence of various impurities in the inhaled air and a decrease in its quality (225-230).

In order for the disease to begin, the pathogen in combination with other factors plays the role of an "ignition system", but with the appearance of a focus of acute pneumonia, the inflammatory process and its effect on the body through a violation of the function of the affected organ come to the fore. Inflammation of the lung tissue means the appearance of new circumstances, which will undoubtedly depend on the localization and volume of the lesion. It is unlikely that anyone will categorically object to the fact that 50% of lung tissue damage is accompanied by a more serious condition of the patient, compared with 5-10%, and that the clinic of lung tissue inflammation will differ from inflammation of the eye or pyelonephritis, regardless of the coincidence of etiology, right? Even a visual representation, which cannot reflect the whole complex of pathophysiological mechanisms arising in AR, allows us to assess the role of the focus of inflammation of the lung tissue for blood circulation in the body (Fig. 2).

From all of the above, the following conclusion logically follows. In order to get out of the web of misconceptions and identify the most important and decisive features of AP for subsequent targeted and successful medical care, there is no other way but a thorough and step-by-step consideration of the factors and mechanisms of disease development in the light of the fundamentals of biomedical science.

4.2.2. Features of the body's reaction to inflammatory damage to lung tissue

Explanations of the clinical diversity of AP today are still largely related to the characteristics of its pathogens, although expert assessments of differential diagnosis even between bacterial and viral forms of the disease do not find fundamental differences and note the extreme difficulty of such separation (116-118). The fact that each case of AP has its own peculiarities and nuances of clinical manifestations is known to every experienced clinician. Such differences in the variants of the individual reaction of the organism to an equivalent stimulus were previously considered as features of reactivity.

Such a reaction of the body has an infinite range of options, which differ, on the one hand, in the speed of development, and, on the other hand, in the level and completeness of adaptation to current changes. Regardless of the final result of such a reaction, its scenario remains stereotypical in all patients with AP, since we are talking about the effect of standard damage to tissue structures, to which each organism reacts individually. However, in the modern interpretation of the mechanisms of AP development, various variants of the causes determining the severity of the patient's condition are presented.

Thus, at present, the nature of the body's reaction to the inflammatory process is no longer considered as features of its reactivity. The latter term is considered insufficiently suitable to describe the phenomena occurring. Now the body's response to any factor causing a general inflammatory reaction is designated as systemic inflammatory reaction syndrome (SIRS), where non-infectious agents can also act as an irritant (169). This term and its defining parameters in relation to various nosologies were aimed at early recognition of patients with sepsis (170,171). However, the automatic inclusion of AP in the cohort of these diseases only led to a further distortion of ideas about the mechanisms of development of this disease.

SIRS as a general reaction of the body is basically a positive phenomenon, which is one of the autonomous forms of its nonspecific protection. However, in the case of a violent reaction of the body, any protective reaction can become uncontrolled and, if methods of its pathogenetic suppression are not applied in a timely manner, this can lead to the development of critical situations. It is these circumstances, combined with a misconception about the sequence of circulatory disorders in patients with AP, from my point of view, can explain the imaginary overdiagnosis of septic complications in them (see above).

In this regard, an important and urgent task is to determine the limits of permissible deviations of SIRS indicators in patients with AP, thanks to which the body is able to resist the action of irritating and damaging factors, while maintaining the necessary functional ability of its vital systems. Currently, the standard mechanisms underlying such a general reaction of the body are known. One of the most important places among these mechanisms is assigned to the production of cytokines. Their increased content was found in the most diverse and incomparable pathological conditions (176,177).

However, interpreting the consequences of the same reaction can lead to completely different conclusions. For example, when the origins of the severity of the condition of patients with AP are analyzed, the initial clinic of the disease is considered as a manifestation of SIRS, but if the situation becomes critical, this syndrome loses its meaning and is replaced by the concept of septic complications accompanied by a cytokine storm. The basics of this paradox have already been discussed in previous sections, but here it is simply necessary to note once again that we are talking about the same reaction of the body with different degrees of severity. In the materials published on this topic, septic (!) complications of AP are declarative in nature without objective evidence of generalization of infection.

Terminology and the concept of the causes of the severe condition of patients with AP in this case are of fundamental importance. Imagine what therapeutic actions should be if we are talking about a rapid deterioration of the patient's condition, but the interpretation of the cause of this crisis may have two incomparable options. In one case, the main mechanism of occurrence of such symptoms is due to the generalization of infection, and in the other, such a picture is explained by a rapid uncompensated violation of the function of the affected organ. Medical care should be aimed at eliminating the cause of the violations that have occurred, which in this case is recognized as the main one, but, depending on the chosen option, it cannot be the same.

The reason for serious misunderstandings is the use of uniform standards for assessing the condition of patients, regardless of the localization of the focus of inflammation. One of the key indicators, which in such assessment systems is considered as a manifestation of septic complications, is arterial hypotension. A decrease in systemic arterial pressure in acute lung tissue damage is a much earlier sign than in pathological processes localized in the vessels of the large circulatory circle. This sign usually accompanies rapidly developing forms of AP, and its appearance in these patients is more a reflection of excessive compensation than a manifestation of sepsis. Therefore, bacteriological blood tests in "septic" patients with AP are usually negative (104, 105).

4.2.3. The main causes of critical situations in acute pneumonia

The modern interpretation of functional disorders resulting from inflammation of the lung tissue focuses on the state of gas exchange, which is considered the main function of the lungs. This implies the process of delivering air to the alveoli and the diffusion of gases. As a result of this emphasis, the cause of respiratory failure is considered to be a violation of ventilation and diffusion in the area of inflammation, although this mechanism does not explain the absence of a strict relationship between the volume of the lesion and the degree of respiratory disorders.

All other functions inherent in the lungs are considered as non-respiratory, and they are not given much importance in the mechanisms of AP. The vascular system of the lungs is considered a blood reservoir, a filter for emboli, a way of transporting vasoactive substances (231-234). Such an important role of small circle vessels as direct participation in the chain of gas exchange and respiration, or regulation of blood flow between two circulatory circles, does not even appear among the mechanisms of functional disorders in AP. Meanwhile, the place and functional significance of pulmonary circulation in the general system of blood flow put forward a violation of its function in the category of the most important pathological mechanisms in AP.

The possibility of early onset of hypotension in patients with aggressive forms of AP, due to the functional features of the pulmonary vessels and their reflex role in the regulation of systemic blood flow, has already been noted above. It should be noted here that the existing conceptual idea of the unlimited influence of the pathogen on the development and features of the manifestations of AP is one of the main reasons for overdiagnosis of septic complications in these patients. These distortions not only affect the diagnosis, but also cause a shift in emphasis in treatment. At the same time, the role of the inflammatory process itself in the mechanisms of the disease remains invisible.

Being an acute inflammatory process, AP shows classic signs of this phenomenon, which inevitably accompany the emerging pathological transformation of the corresponding tissue structures. The appearance of these signs is an integral accompaniment of inflammatory processes, regardless of our attention to them and our assessment of these characteristics. Described many centuries ago by Celsus and Galen, these distinctive features of inflamed tissues (heat, pain, redness, swelling and loss of function) have passed the test of time and remain an important link of our fundamental knowledge in the section of inflammatory diseases (90,154).

The existing classics of the development of inflammation obliges us to take into account the role and significance of each of the manifestations of this process in the formation of the overall picture of the disease. The described signs of inflammation have a close and inextricable connection with each other, since they reflect one common phenomenon, however, the first four characteristics of the inflammatory process (heat, pain, redness, swelling) are more local. Given the deep localization of the focus of inflammation in AP, signs such as redness and swelling can only be detected and confirmed by special studies. For example, when performing chest radiography, the focus of inflammation receives a specific image due to its excessive blood filling, edema and tissue infiltration.

Pain in acute inflammation is the result of changes in the biochemical composition of tissues and irritation of sensitive receptors. However, it is known that pain syndrome in patients with AP occurs only if pleural leaves are involved in the process. In most patients, the development of a focus of inflammation in the lung is not accompanied by pain, since pain receptors are absent inside this organ and are located only on its external borders (154). In this regard, it should be noted that the causes causing the pain reaction can be an irritant for other tissue structures, including nerve receptors with other functions.

The most important sign of inflammation from a clinical point of view is a violation of the function of the affected organ. It is this sign that reflects the features of the clinical picture of the disease, depending on the functional significance of the affected organ for the whole organism. In this regard, it is impossible to make a mistake comparing inflammation of the middle ear with panaritium or conjunctivitis with arthritis of the ankle joint. These examples, which at first glance may seem inappropriate and too revealing, are not given by chance, since such comparisons should help to understand how wrong it is to compare some critical manifestations of AP with similar signs in other inflammatory processes.

It is the comparison of critical situations in the clinic of various diseases, when their features begin to manifest themselves most expressively, that makes it easier and more complete to get an idea of the specifics of their mechanisms. However, currently septic complications of inflammatory processes are evaluated and analyzed according to the same scheme, regardless of the diagnosis (82-86,105). In such analytical materials, patients with AP are not separated into a separate group and are considered by analogy with other variants of inflammatory processes. At the same time, these patients account for up to 40-50% of the total number of cases with septic complications (25).

In the modern concept of AP, the cause of respiratory failure in these patients is mainly considered to be a violation of the diffusion of gases in the alveoli due to the loss of air permeability by the lung tissue as a result of edema and inflammatory infiltration (155-158, 174). But, it must be remembered that gas exchange in the body is represented by a sequential chain of mechanisms that begins with the inhalation of outdoor air and ends with the delivery of gases to the tissues of the body. This pathway acts in two opposite directions, providing the main goal of gas exchange, its maintenance at the cellular level.

It is quite obvious that the loss of any link from the general "route" will be accompanied by a clinic of respiratory disorders and, in addition to alveolar diffusion, general blood flow disorders accompanying aggressive forms of the disease will inevitably play a negative role in this general process. It was found that as a result of inflammatory transformation, the lung tissue loses its elasticity, however, the study of this characteristic does not reveal a direct relationship between the volume of the lesion and the degree of respiratory disorders, thereby showing that alveolar diffusion disorder is not the only and main factor of respiratory failure (158,159).

When studying the causes of respiratory failure in patients with distress syndrome, the involvement of the lungs in blood circulation is mentioned only indirectly in connection with the analysis of gas diffusion disorders and a decrease in blood oxygenation. Inhomogeneity of lung perfusion and shunting of part of the blood through unventilated parts of the organ is usually noted (155,156). Such an assessment of pulmonary perfusion shifts as an additional mechanism of respiratory failure is explained by the fact that the purpose of the study is not aimed at clarifying the causes and sequence of disorders, but at finding optimal options for auxiliary care for these patients when performing lung ventilation. The authors do not hide that the purpose of the study is to solve this purely palliative problem (157,159,160).

The reason for such a one-sided study of the mechanisms of AP is still the fixation of attention exclusively on the etiology of the disease. The influence of the pathogen on the characteristics of respiratory dysfunction continues to dominate the scientific worldview as the main reason for the peculiarities of clinical manifestations. For example, S-Y.Ruan et al. (161) analyzed the distress syndrome in patients with AP depending on the etiology, trying to find such features. Having found no differences in this form of lung damage between bacterial and viral processes, the authors consider it necessary to continue such searches.

Examples like the one above show what a deep mark a long period of excessive hopes for the exclusive role of antibiotics has left in the modern professional worldview. Today, the main research and searches are aimed at identifying new etiotropic approaches to neutralizing the pathogens of AP or the results of their action. Meanwhile, it should be noted that in the above-mentioned work

(161), the authors conducted a fairly detailed analysis and obtained the corresponding result. This result, contrary to assumptions, turned out to be negative, but it showed that there are no fundamental (!) differences in this direction. The repetition or continuation of such a search should be discussed only if the initial analytical work was carried out with identified violations and deviations, right?

Similar examples are found in large numbers in modern publications today, since many researchers focus only on the expected result and on this basis believe that the study has not achieved its goal. And if we look at this problem from a different point of view and question the legitimacy and infallibility of the chosen goal? A negative result of the conducted research is a completely reasonable result and, if there is no doubt about the usefulness of the search, then such a final should be evaluated properly.

All the last remarks are not a departure from the topic discussed in this section, but on the contrary, they are another prerequisite for understanding the reasons for forgetting some fundamental scientific materials. Therefore, continuing the discussion of functional disorders in acute inflammation of the lung tissue, it is impossible to ignore the features of pulmonary blood flow, its role in the regulation of systemic circulation and their close interdependence.

In order to pay attention to the missing features of pulmonary functions in the existing assessments of the mechanisms of AP development, it is necessary to recall basic medical information on this topic, which is included in the general education programs of medical universities. The human circulatory system is divided into two circuits that are inextricably linked both anatomically and functionally. However, the purpose of providing vital functions has different meanings for the large and small circulatory circles. This is reflected both in the features of their anatomical structure and in the functional parameters.

Blood pressure in the pulmonary vessels is about 5-8 times lower than systemic arterial pressure, and its increase by only 5-10 mmHg can lead to pulmonary tissue edema (101,162). To avoid such a dangerous situation for the body, nature has provided for the presence of baroreceptors in the pulmonary vessels, the irritation of which is accompanied by a decrease in venous return and unloading of the small circle as a result of a decrease in peripheral blood pressure. In this case, we are talking about the above-mentioned Schwiegk's reflex, which has been known for almost a hundred years since its first description (91). This mechanism also reduces the cardiac load and facilitates the synchronous work of the two halves of the cardiovascular system.

The inflammatory vascular reaction already at the initial stages of the pathological process is accompanied by a change in blood flow parameters with the participation of pulmonary vascular baroreceptors. An increase in blood flow to the area of inflammation, followed by a slowdown in blood flow in this segment of the circulation, leads to an increase in intravascular pressure and the reaction of baroreceptors. However, in this situation, the manifestation of circulatory disorders and regulatory lung function will depend on the individual combinations between the rate of development of the inflammatory process and the compensatory and adaptive capabilities of the body. The range of such combinations is infinite, which is one of our individual characteristics.

In the case of a relatively slow development of the inflammatory process, the body has enough time to adapt to disorders of pulmonary circulation. If the pressure in the vessels of the small circle increases gradually, the body manages to deposit part of the circulating blood relatively unnoticeably, reducing the load on the pulmonary bed and preventing the occurrence of a critical situation.

The scenario of the development of the inflammatory process in AP is standard for this nosological form. However, in the case of aggressive development of the disease, the ability to adapt is significantly reduced, since the body must perform compensatory reactions at a speed adequate to the rapid dynamics of inflammation. As a result of the fact that the body of many patients does not have time to adapt the synchronicity of its circulatory system to unexpected and rapidly progressive violations of its parameters, there are increasing signs of pathological functional shifts.

Today, an important characteristic that is constantly taken into account when assessing the condition of patients with AP is the indicator of systemic blood pressure. This indicator is accepted as one of the main ones in the existing methods for determining the severity of the course of the disease (126-129). The fundamental misconception in this case is the fact that in patients with AP it is necessary to evaluate and correct blood flow disorders in the pulmonary vessels. After all, it is the vessels of the small circle of blood circulation that are the primary link in the chain of vascular mechanisms in AP.

Peripheral circulatory disorders in patients with AP are primarily the result of compensatory shifts, which play a secondary, rather than a leading role in the pathogenesis of the disease. With the help of such deviations, the body strives to adapt the work of its cardiovascular system to suddenly emerging new conditions. Therefore, the correction of such disorders, especially in the initial period of the disease, is able to disrupt the adaptation process to a greater extent. At the same time, the place of the main cause of such deviations is assigned to the causative agent of the process, while the influence of inflamed areas of the lungs on their functional state, as the true root cause, is not given importance. Such a modern version of assessments and further treatment is not even accompanied by references to the existing relationship between the two circulatory circles and the mechanisms of their interaction and regulation.

Modern interpretations of the mechanisms of AP and the search for solutions to this problem do not take into account the differences between the small and large circulatory circles. The concept of the disease is still based on the etiology of the process, but the properties of pathogens can be studied in detail only in laboratory conditions. The influence of pathogens on the clinical picture in a real situation, when they face multifactorial protection of a living organism, is presented in the form of analogies with laboratory data, which are used as virtual explanations and assumptions. The collapse of versatile and numerous attempts at differential diagnosis of AP in accordance with its etiology is a convincing confirmation of the fact that the exact effect of each pathogen on the clinic and features of AP remains uncertain, and laboratory differences of pathogens are not accompanied by the same obvious clinical discrepancies.

If we focus on modern interpretations of the mechanisms of the disease, they do not take into account the difference between small and large circulatory circles, and the search for a solution to the problem goes without taking this factor into account. The concept of disease is still based on a microbiological foundation. The properties of pathogens studied in laboratory conditions of the greenhouse are used for virtual explanations of the development of pathological conditions. How the qualities of pathogens manifest themselves in a real situation when they encounter multifactorial resistance of a living organism remains precisely unknown. Descriptions of the results of the action of individual pathogens on body tissues are based on analogies and assumptions, since such consequences of excessive protective reactions are an almost untouched topic.

Considering the modern interpretation of the causes of circulatory disorders observed in patients with AP, it is impossible to ignore the fact that the classical physiology of the circulatory system has almost completely lost its presence in the concept of the disease. The ideology of the AP tries to balance on a narrow platform of microbiological causes of the process. Therefore, when patients with AP have a decrease in peripheral blood pressure, it is considered as the development of septic complications as a result of generalization of infection (85,86).

Assessing the cause of the decrease in peripheral blood pressure in patients with AP as a result of sepsis and septic shock, the fact that in most cases in this particular group microbiological blood examination does not confirm the septic nature of complications has ceased to be taken into account (104,105). The desire to focus on the infectious nature of the disease is the reason for the rather strange and not entirely logical explanations for such negative tests. For example, the absence of pathogenic microorganisms in the blood is explained by preliminary antibacterial therapy (102-104), leaving open the question of how septic complications arose with such effective treatment?

If among patients with bacterial forms of AP, blood cultures with sepsis and septic shock reveal the causative agent in at least a small number of observations (87.88), then with viral pneumonia, the presence of viruses in the general bloodstream and their role in septic complications have no objective evidence at all. The diagnosis of septic complications of viral infection is exclusively declarative and is approved on the basis of clinical analogies with the traditions of assessing bacterial pneumonia. Nasopharyngeal smears confirming the presence of COVID-19 viral infection cannot serve as an argument in favor of septic complications, since such tests are characteristic of all cases of infection and do not reflect the generalization of the infectious onset (82.83).

A feature of modern clinical studies of septic complications of viral forms of AP are attempts to find ways to neutralize the causes of their development and eliminate their manifestations. And since the causative agent of the process itself is recognized as the main cause of the disease, against which no effective means have been found in such observations, the attention of researchers is focused on the general manifestations of generalized infection, regardless of the localization of the focus of inflammation and the functional significance of the affected organ.

Currently, due to the appearance of a large group of patients with COVID-19 pneumonia who are deprived of traditional etiotropic treatment, interest in additional methods of medical care has increased. One of the most serious and tragic causes of the severity of the disease is considered to be a sharp increase in cytokine production, which is designated by the term "cytokine storm" (176-178). It was during the pandemic that interest in eliminating this phenomenon increased, which, according to many experts, can significantly improve the results of treatment of this group of patients (179-184).

At the same time, it is known that an increase in the level of cytokines in the blood is not a sign specific to pneumonia, and can be observed in situations not related to inflammation or infection at all (176-178). It is also known that cytokines are one of the forms of a non-specific reaction of the body to various stimuli, play the role of immunomodulatory factors and have many varieties with a variety of their functions. The information already known to date about the importance of cytokines for the body allows us to identify these factors as protective and adaptive, which initially have the image of a positive phenomenon. However, as is already known by the example of other compensatory mechanisms, such reactions can exceed the limit of their useful effect, which leads to negative consequences.

In recent years, the role of cytokines in the development of pathological processes and, in particular, in AP has been investigated. The mechanisms of inflammatory diseases have remained the same, but now there is an idea of what is happening at the moment at the cellular and molecular level. The discovery and study of the role of cytokines in the development of the disease does not mean at all that these substances are the factor, eliminating which, you can count on a win-win success of treatment. They are the result and consequence of the influence of other causes, are not necessarily associated with inflammation or infection and, as is known, do not directly depend on the etiology. Being a reflection of one of the compensatory-adaptive reactions of the body, cytokines, like many protective reactions, can take the form of an uncontrolled process that turns into a serious problem.

During the development of the disease, various changes and deviations can occur in the body, which have a causal relationship with each other. In the process of studying such conditions, our knowledge and ideas are supplemented with information about current processes at the level of cells and molecules, but this information does not change the origin of clinical symptoms. Therefore, the expansion of horizons in a certain direction does not at all mean a mandatory guide to action. In this regard, it is necessary to recall the old postulate of medicine that there is a so-called norm in pathology. That is, it is thanks to the resulting deviations of various constants of the organism that the latter has the ability to withstand a sudden catastrophe. As an example and comparison with a cytokine storm, the following well-known information can be cited.

One of the signs of inflammatory or infectious processes is an increase in body temperature. In such situations, leukocytes secrete pyrogens that act on the anterior hypothalamus, which is responsible for thermoregulation (185). An increase in body temperature stimulates many protective functions of the body, reflecting its ability to resist. In particular, some options for treating cancer patients by purposefully increasing body temperature are based on these principles (186). However, prolonged, excessive and uncontrolled increase in temperature leads to the development of hyperthermia, which already poses a danger to the patient's life. For example, about half a million patients die from hyperthermia every year in the world (185).

Hyperthermia has been known to medicine for much longer than information about the cytokine storm. Nevertheless, as you know, no one has tried to solve the problem of certain diseases by normalizing the elevated temperature. In this regard, only the task of preventing the transition of the temperature reaction into hyperthermic syndrome, thereby preventing unforeseen critical complications was solved. Normalization of temperature in patients with inflammation is not at all equivalent to their cure, is it? It seems to me that this is the meaning of the cytokine storm, and in this aspect it is necessary to decide by virtue of what therapeutic omissions it arose and what are the origins of its occurrence. To develop the idea of simple neutralization of cytokines is too primitive and short-sighted.

A somewhat more detailed consideration of the cytokine storm was taken only as an example from a whole series of similar narrowly focused studies. Currently, as a rule, one of the manifestations of AP with an attempt to achieve positive clinical results is taken as the goal of the study. Such studies have been particularly intensified recently in connection with the coronavirus pandemic and the loss of the role of antibiotics. Among the mosaic of studies of individual manifestations of COVID-19 pneumonia, along with cytokines, the value of angiotensin receptor blockers is being clarified (187-192), the most beneficial combinations of immunomodulators are being actively studied (193-197) and, of course, retesting of already known antiviral and anti-inflammatory drugs is being carried out (37,43,44,117,149,181,182,198-200).

A common feature of all such studies is the choice of one of the links in the pathogenesis of the disease as the main goal. Such principles of studying the problem of AP can explain the fact that among the huge number of publications devoted to this topic, it is impossible to single out works whose results reflect a real step forward in solving it and which would already differ in certain practical achievements.

The only way to treat patients with COVID-19 pneumonia, the use of which gives a slight and not always convincing improvement in their condition, is to turn to hormone therapy (201-208). However, this type of medical care, as is well known, has long been used in situations where there is no clear understanding of the causes of the severity of the condition of patients and ways to effectively support them in such a situation. Hormones in such circumstances act as an anti-stress agent. The logic of the narrow research projects carried out today, from my point of view, can only be explained by the strong dependence of scientific research on the stereotypes of recent decades. After all, even in the absence of the expected positive results, most authors of such works remain convinced supporters of continuing their searches.

4.2.4. Acute pneumonia is more of a circulatory than a respiratory catastrophe

If we now return to the question of the interdependence and regulation of blood flow between the two circulatory circles, then the clinical picture of severe forms of AP, which today is considered as sepsis or septic shock, may appear in a completely different perspective.

The onset of an inflammatory reaction is accompanied by the mobilization of the body's defenses. One of these standard reactions is the stage of arterial hyperemia with increased blood flow to this area for the delivery of cellular and humoral protection factors. An unexpected and rapid increase in blood filling of the pulmonary vessels inevitably leads to irritation of their baroreceptors regulating systemic arterial pressure and circulating blood volume (235-237).

Aggressive development of inflammation in the lung tissue increases the pressure in the vessels of the small circle, but the body does not have time to deposit part of the circulating blood in such conditions. To relieve the pulmonary vessels and reduce the risk of subsequent pulmonary edema, an emergency mechanism is activated, which works almost instantly. In such situations, there is a reflex decrease in the tone of peripheral vessels with an increase in the capacity of the large circulatory circle and the diversion of part of the blood to the periphery.

In the clinical picture, such situations are manifested by hypotension, and in the most severe cases, a violation of tissue perfusion at the periphery proceeds with a typical picture of shock. In such a situation, shock is a consequence of a violation of pulmonary circulation, and not of septic origin and deserves its designation as pulmonogenic (163). Subsequent multiple organ failure is the result of impaired perfusion of various organs and tissues with a violation of their nutrition and metabolism (164,165). However, today most explanations of the cause of these complications are based, like the shock that preceded them, on an infectious origin (25,166). A significant difference in shockogenic factors determines different approaches to their elimination, therefore, determining the causes of shock in patients with AP is not an idle occupation at all.

Now, when patients with AP are diagnosed with sepsis and septic shock, this implies intravenous infusions (in the form of boluses) to replenish the volume of circulating blood and eliminate hypotension (25,82,86,105,125,172). However, this therapeutic procedure is directed against the compensatory reaction in AP, since, contrary to the body's desire to unload the pulmonary vessels, intravenous infusions, on the contrary, support and increase blood flow (see Figure 3). Despite the confident tone of such recommendations on the use of intravenous infusions for AP, they are accompanied in advance by an indirect recognition of their frequent inefficiency, which is expressed in urgent advice not to postpone the use of vasopressors if resuscitation with fluid does not bring a quick effect (6.82 105 173).

If we take into account that these therapeutic measures are used in the most severe patients with AP hospitalized in intensive care units, then the effectiveness of such care is expressed in its results. And the results speak for themselves - mortality among patients with AP in the intensive care unit in recent years is 30-50% (21-29, 167), and in septic (?) shock can reach 91% (168).

But not only the results give a serious reason for an in-depth analysis of the causes that destroy the efforts of modern medicine to change the current situation. It is impossible not to pay attention to the frank confessions of some authors that the condition of many patients continues to deteriorate after hospitalization (158). Even more disturbing are the sincere statements that the overwhelming number of patients with septic shock did not have it during hospitalization (!) and it developed during treatment (85). Such revelations can appear only on the basis of their own experience and indirectly indicate the shortcomings of treatment. This fully corresponds to the old rule of medicine that if the patient's condition does not improve after the start of treatment, then this treatment does not correspond to this disease.

In this regard, it should be noted that the cause of obstruction of blood flow in the small circle of circulation, which begins the chain of mechanisms that ultimately lead to the picture of shock, is a generalized spasm of the pulmonary vessels in response to irritation emanating from the focus of inflammation. This statement is based on objective evidence of reflex action of the affected area on the entire pool of pulmonary vessels.

In the course of the above-mentioned research work (135), one of its fragments was the study of the effectiveness of certain medical procedures and, in particular, cervical vagosympathetic blockade (CVSB). The blockade technique was developed and described by A.A.Vishnevsky in 1932. This type of blockade was allowed for clinical use and became widespread in the Soviet Union, where this work was carried out. CVSB was, in particular, recommended for the differential diagnosis of abdominal pain syndrome in AP and acute appendicitis in children. Even before the start of these studies, when performing the blockade for diagnostic purposes, attention was paid to a noticeable improvement in the condition and well-being of patients if the cause of their disease was due to AP.

The results obtained should be presented here when discussing this issue, and so that they do not look nameless, a brief description of the technique of this blockade is provided. The patient lies on his back with a small roller under the shoulder blades. The head is thrown back and turned in the opposite direction from the blockade. The patient's arm is slightly lowered along the body from the side of the procedure.

The doctor places the index finger of the left hand just above the intersection point of the external jugular vein with the posterior edge of the sternocleidomastoid muscle. By pressing this point, the doctor medially shifts the muscles and blood vessels and feels the anterior surface of the cervical vertebrae. The needle is inserted near the tip of the finger and directed to the front surface of the cervical vertebrae. When the tip of the needle rests against the anterior surface of the vertebra, the needle is slightly pulled, a trial aspiration is performed to make sure that there is no puncture of the vessel, and then an anesthetic solution is injected. The dose of 0.25% novocaine solution in children ranges from 5 to 15 ml, depending on age, in adult patients up to 30-60 ml. The anesthetic solution blocks the vagus and sympathetic nerves. Gorner's syndrome (ptosis, miosis, enophthalmos), which appears literally within 2-5 minutes, is an indicator of the effectiveness of the blockade.

An objective assessment of the effect of this procedure on the functional parameters of the pulmonary-cardiac apparatus was carried out using comparative rheopulmonography (CRPG). The initial registration of indicators was carried out immediately before the procedure, and then immediately after its completion. The recording electrodes were located on the side wall of the chest at the level of 3-4 ribs and they remained in the same place until the indicators were re-registered. The recording was made on the Elkar RPG-4 unit (USSR). The CRPG study was conducted in 22 patients with CVSB. The age of the patients in these studies ranged from 3.5 to 14 years.

CRPG allowed to estimate respiratory rate (RR), respiratory volume (RV), minute ventilation volume (MV), heart rate (HR), systolic wave amplitude (SA), minute pulsating blood flow (MBF), ventilation and perfusion ratio (K v/p). Statistical processing of the materials was carried out using unique abbreviated methods, which were noted above when evaluating the results of experimental studies (137).

The results of CRPG were an objective confirmation of the effect of CVSB in patients with AP. The initial indicators indicated a pronounced predominance of ventilation parameters over the indicators of blood flow in the lung tissue. When analyzing the data obtained after the procedure, there was a significant decrease ($p=0.001$) in the parameters MV, RR, MBF and SA. After the treatment procedures, the ratio between the parameters of ventilation and blood flow (K v/p) leveled off. These changes were accompanied by a noticeable improvement in the general condition and well-being of patients.

A decrease in the capacity of the small circle and a relative excess of venous return is the reason for an increase in respiratory excursions, which have a massaging effect on the lungs. As a result, ventilation indicators begin to grow relative to blood flow parameters. However, such a shift does not improve blood oxygen saturation, since the amount of blood passing through the narrowed microvessels of the lungs remains low. Performing CVSB eliminates the reflex effect of the focus of inflammation on the vascular bed of the small circle in the intact parts of the lungs, and this effect can be recorded within a few minutes after the procedure. The control record of the CRPG showed a decrease in enhanced ventilation and relief of pulmonary blood flow with an equalization of the proportions between them and a subsequent increase in blood oxygen saturation.

The presence of such reflex dependence and its role in the pathogenesis of AP can be clearly demonstrated using comparative rheopulmonograms recorded before and after cervical vagosympathetic novocaine blockade (Fig. 12-13).

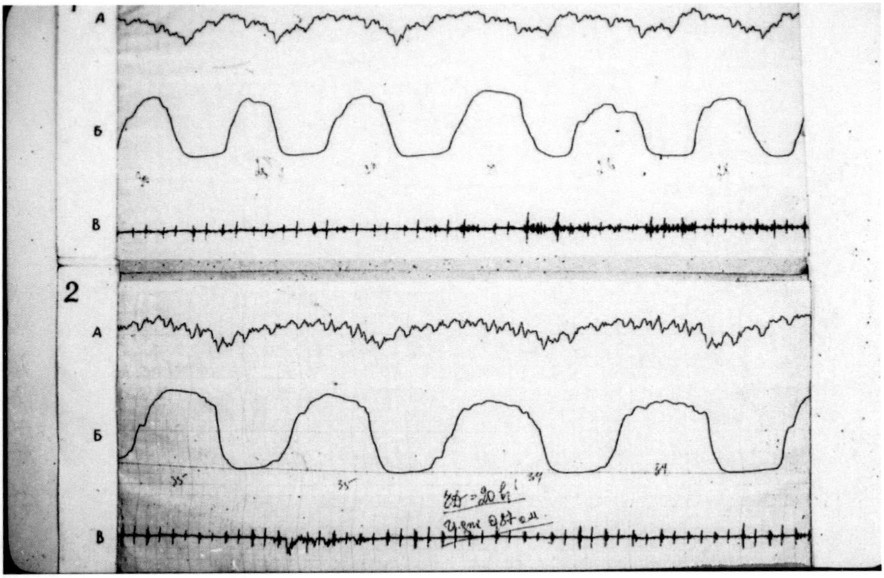

Figure 12. Rheogram of ventilation of the patient 8 years old, AP 7-10 segments of the right lung.

1-the original reopulmonography (RPG).

2-RPG after vagosympathetic blockade

A-differential RPGs

Б-Main RPG

B-phonocardiogram

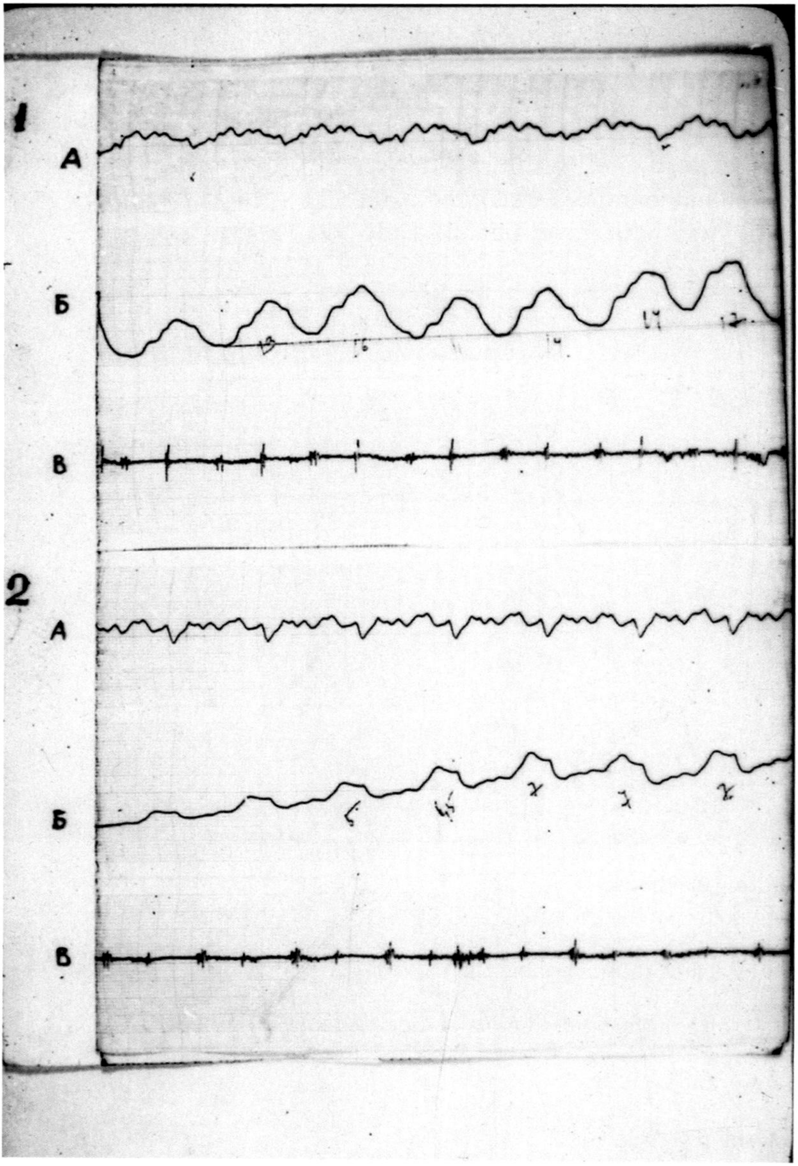

Figure 13. Rheogram of pulsatory blood flow of the same patient. The designations are the same.

It is quite acceptable that the RPG recordings presented today look somewhat primitive against the background of modern research capabilities. However, despite the fact that this information was received more than 30 years ago, I am deeply convinced that it has not lost its significance. Moreover, in the light of modern ideas about the mechanisms of AP development based on impressions, assumptions and analogies with other inflammatory processes, these data favorably differ in their objective characteristics and can serve as a basis for more in-depth studies.

Currently, among the many publications with information on the problem under discussion, there are individual messages that stand out with non-standard material and, at the same time, serve as additional arguments in favor of the above interpretation of vascular disorders in AP. For example, M.Thillai et al. noted that hypoxemia in patients with COVID-19 pneumonia does not correspond to the condition of the lungs on radiographs. After determining the volume of blood in the lungs using tomography, the authors found a significant decrease in blood flow in small vessels up to 2 mm in diameter and concluded that this phenomenon is due to their spasm or thrombosis (93). Such generalized thrombosis in this segment of the circulatory system is hardly compatible with life, but the spastic state of these vessels fully explains the observed functional disorders.

In another message, the author drew attention to the fact that patients with COVID-19 pneumonia who received captopril to reduce systemic blood pressure cope with the disease much easier and faster (175). Unfortunately, the author does not give his version of such an effect, but the mechanism of this phenomenon, from my point of view, is quite clear. The drug reduces the tone of peripheral vessels and thereby increases the capacity of the large circle of blood circulation, reducing venous return and unloading the small circle.

Publications like the above examples are rare, since the materials underlying them are not the result of purposeful research and, most likely, are in the nature of unexpected findings, the authors of which find it difficult to interpret them. The vast majority of research conducted today is aimed at finding means to neutralize the causative agent of the disease and eliminate the consequences of its activities. Such a specific, but narrow formulation of the goal leads to a clear simplification of the pathogenesis of the disease with the loss of causal relationships in the chain of mechanisms of the process.

The development of circulatory disorders in AP is interpreted as a result of generalized infection, therefore, the choice of means of suppressing the pathogen when signs resembling sepsis and septic shock appear in patients with this disease is currently the main task of treatment. Such a system of views on this pathology leaves aside scientific information about the features of the small circle of blood circulation and its role in the regulation of systemic blood flow.

The recommendations and directives resulting from this AP concept, similar to the principles of medical care for septic complications of other diseases, actually represent, especially at the early stages of the process in the lungs, counteraction to compensatory reactions of the body. The fictitious frequency of septic complications in lung tissue inflammation is emphasized by negative microbiological tests and, most importantly, the results of such care.

4.2.5. Fundamentals of pathological transformation of tissues in the focus of inflammation

If general and systemic changes in blood circulation determine the severity of AP, then the features of the restructuring of blood flow in the area of inflammation determine the depth of tissue damage. Increasing edema and infiltration of tissues in the area of inflammation can create a "vascular trap" mechanism, when there is a compression of more malleable blood outflow routes against the background of its preserved or even increased inflow. With the preserved dynamics of the development of this mechanism, it is possible to stop blood flow with further trophic disruption and tissue necrosis. Examples and evidence of such a vascular mechanism in AP have been presented in the previous sections.

In the latter case, we are talking about postmortem contrast of lung vessels, which allowed us to see the features of lung angioarchitectonics in AP. Unfortunately, these studies gave an answer to one of the questions posed, showing only the vascular network of the small circle. The second source of blood supply to the bronchopulmonary system remained unexplored. In the available literature, we could not find reliable facts about which structures of the lung tissue the inflammatory reaction begins. Although the method of obtaining such information seems very complicated, meanwhile it could explain the variants of the development of the inflammatory process in the lungs.

The starting point of the inflammatory reaction would be important in light of the fact that the blood supply to the lungs comes from two sources. Bronchial structures up to the bronchioles receive blood supply from the bronchial arteries, which belong to a large circle of blood circulation and originate from the aortic arch. Parenchymal parts of the organ are provided with blood flowing in the vessels of the small circle. There is a connection between two blood supply systems in the form of shunts that can function in certain situations (234, 238-240).

The role of bronchial vessels, which have an anatomical connection with the vessels of the lungs through shunts, but differ from them by significantly higher blood pressure, requires study in the mechanism of inflammatory vascular reaction in AP. This anatomical feature may have an impact on the variant of the development of the inflammatory process. If the inflammatory process originates in the alveolar parts of the lung, then the vascular reaction and subsequent hyperemia of this zone will be associated only with the pulmonary vessels. In this case, the dynamics of the focus of inflammation will resemble a "blurred spot", as this phenomenon was described in the old literature.

If we assume that acute inflammation begins in the bronchial structures, then the vascular reaction and sudden blood flow occur in the bronchial artery basin. Under these conditions, blood from the zone with higher pressure can be discharged through shunts into the vessels of the small circle, disrupting blood flow in them. In the case of an aggressive development of events, such a mechanism for the spread of primary affect can lead to a sudden and rapid overflow of the vascular bed of entire segments or lobes of the lung, manifested by the so-called croup form of pneumonia.

The described variants of the development of the AP focus are nothing more than an assumption, although they are based on well-known features of the blood supply to the lung tissue and clinical and radiological manifestations of the disease. The reality of such a mechanism of lobar forms of AP, from my point of view, is very likely, but requires additional research and evidence. During the period of research on this topic, we did not have the technical capabilities to verify these assumptions at least at the level of a postmortem study of angioarchitectonics. However, the results of such a study will be important for understanding the causes of the development of large-volume lung tissue lesions, including total lung necrosis, which has already been noted with a new variant of COVID-19 pneumonia (241,242).

The development of necrotic changes in the pulmonary parenchyma in AP is an irreversible stage of the process and in most cases, especially with a small area of damage, is accompanied by lysis of non-viable tissues, further cleaning of this area and its replacement with new tissue. However, this option is the most favorable, but, unfortunately, sometimes the necrosis zone is cleared with the appearance of new problems. The emergence of new clinical and radiological situations depends on a number of factors.

When such a defect is localized in the deep layers of the organ, sufficiently large necrosis zones in the case of emptying through the adductor bronchus are able to position themselves as cavities. At the same time, the radiological signs of such destruction cavities will depend on the diameter and patency of the draining bronchi. Complete evacuation of detritus and preservation of the bronchial lumen is accompanied by the appearance of irregularly shaped cavities on radiographs, the walls of which can contour due to the remaining perifocal inflammation.

Incomplete evacuation of the contents from the destruction zone leads to the appearance of cavities with a liquid level. This picture is a classic example of the formation of an abscess in the lung, and, as a rule, the purulent nature of its internal accumulation makes it necessary to solve new tactical problems during treatment.

Bronchitis in the adducting bronchi can reduce their drainage capabilities, which is reflected in the diagnostic signs of necrotic cavities. Narrowing of the bronchial lumen is one of the factors of abscess formation. Partial blockade of the bronchi with the development of a valve mechanism in their lumen can lead to an increase in the diameter of such cavities as a result of excess air retention in them. A sign of such cavities on radiographs is, according to the laws of physics, a clear circle shape due to an increase in internal pressure. Necrosis zones located in the superficial parts of the lungs can bring much more serious troubles, but these options will be discussed in the corresponding section below.

Necrotic lesions of large lung tissue deserve special attention. In this case, we are talking about a total lesion of the lung lobe or even the entire lung. Such forms of organ tissue damage create a situation that, in the case of wait-and-see tactics, leads to an inevitable fatal outcome. The volume of the lesion leaves no hope that the patient's body will be able to independently (even against the background of intensive medical support) remove a huge array of non-viable tissues without accompanying fatal complications. Fortunately, such forms of lesion are quite rare, but their development does not change depending on the etiological dynamics of AP. Total necrotic pneumonia of the lung lobe (gangrene) was observed with bacterial inflammation and continues to occur with viral lesion (241,242,282-284).

4.2.6. Violation of bronchial patency

Taking into account the peculiarities of changes in blood flow in the pulmonary vessels in AP, it is impossible to ignore such an important sign of the disease as the loss of airiness by the lung tissue and the causes of this phenomenon. The disappearance of air from the alveolar parts of the organ is caused not only by their filling with inflammatory exudate, but also by the blockade of the corresponding bronchial branches. The latter circumstance disrupts ventilation and bronchial drainage of the attached parenchyma of the organ and is an explanation for the fact that insufficiently active recanalization of the respiratory tract in the area of inflammation slows down the elimination of this pathological transformation.

The cause of bronchial patency disorder is endobronchial inflammation, the clinical signs of which often precede the development of AP. Bronchitis and bronchiolitis are accompanied by swelling of the mucous membrane, excessive mucus secretion and spasm of bronchial muscles. In addition to these endobronchial factors, compression of small bronchial branches by the inflammatory infiltrate surrounding them is added.

As the diameter of the bronchi decreases, they gradually lose their cartilaginous framework and lose the ability to constantly maintain their lumen, following the example of the trachea or large bronchi. In the same sequence, the relative volume of muscles in the bronchial wall increases, increasing the value of bronchospasm among obstructive factors. Consequently, the smaller the diameter of the bronchial branches, the easier it is to disrupt their lumen. At the same time, the difficulty of recanalization of the airways in severe situations increases inversely in proportion to their size.

In conditions of endobronchitis and accumulation of secretions in the lumen of the bronchi, the mucociliary apparatus cannot provide the necessary cleaning of their lumen and such a protective mechanism as cough is included in this process (247,248). It is with the help of cough that the body is able to remove excess contents from the bronchial tree. However, this protective mechanism is most active in the upper respiratory tract. The cough reflex is most sensitive in the larynx and trachea, gradually decreasing in the direction of deepening into the lungs. The air flow velocity during a cough, which determines its performance, is maximal in the larynx, where it can reach 100 miles per hour (247). The smallest branches of the bronchial tree, which are more clogged, are in the most unfavorable position to release their lumen.

It should be noted that in modern clinical practice, chronic bronchitis occupies a special place in respiratory pathology. At the same time, in patients with AP who had no breathing problems before the disease, signs of concomitant bronchitis are usually not given much importance, since the attention of attending physicians is focused on the focus of inflammation in the lung and its probable causative agent. Inflammatory changes in the bronchi in such patients are regarded as a consequence of the infectious factor AP, and their elimination is provided by etiotropic therapy. The presence of bronchitis in AP is described as an accumulation of secretions in the bronchi and is only rarely noted by clinicians or even pathologists (249-252).

In bacterial forms of AP, the presence of cough and sputum discharge in patients is one of the most pathognomonic signs of the disease. The cause of these manifestations is endobronchitis, but the degree of bronchial obstruction in different parts of the lungs varies markedly. In such observations, we conducted two variants of the study of bronchial patency.

Firstly, as noted above, in the initial period of work, we performed microtracheostomy contrast after its superposition in order to determine the localization of its distal (internal) end. A total of 44 such studies were conducted. During the performance of such studies, a contrast agent was observed to enter the distal parts of the bronchial tree, which in these patients constantly demonstrated the blocking of branches in the focus of inflammation. An illustration of such a study was presented in Chapter 3 (see section 3.2.2 Figure 8).

Secondly, a contrast study of the bronchial tree was conducted on 9 lung preparations taken from children who died from AP. The results of these studies were also presented in chapter 3 (see section 3.2.2 Figure 7). In all cases, there was no penetration of contrast into the bronchi in the area of inflammation, which was associated with the blockade of these branches.

The dynamics of the etiology of AP, which has been observed in recent decades, did not significantly affect the main signs of the disease. For example, the recent increase in the number of patients with lung damage by coronavirus has not removed from the agenda the issue of bronchial patency disorders in such observations (251, 252). Morphological postmortem studies of the bronchopulmonary apparatus after coronavirus damage show almost constant detection of bronchitis phenomena (285). However, confirmation of signs of endobronchitis and bronchial lumen disorders in COVID-19 pneumonia is not reflected in the principles of treatment.

Modern recommendations for helping patients with AP include attempts to neutralize various manifestations of the inflammatory process at the cellular and molecular level, but methods of bronchial recanalization and restoration of ventilation of affected areas of lung tissue are not actually included in the modern treatment package. Some reports indicate the positive effect of drugs that dilute bronchial secretions (250,253-256). However, in the recommendations for the use of these drugs, which play a passive role in the process of recanalization of the bronchial lumen, more importance is attached to their possible antibacterial and antiviral properties. Thus, we are talking about strengthening etiotropic therapy, and not about restoring bronchial patency.

The exclusively passive effect of sputum dilution drugs on the restoration of bronchial patency is demonstrated by the lack of effect from their use at critical stages of the disease, when the ability of patients to actively remove sputum is sharply reduced or simply absent (257). The vagueness of ideas about the mechanisms and significance of bronchial blockade in AR, as well as the role of cough as an important protective mechanism, is confirmed by such a fact as the ongoing discussion about the use of drugs to suppress the cough reflex in patients with signs of bronchitis (258-261).

Is it any wonder that in recent years the consequences of transferred inflammatory processes in bronchopulmonary structures have become more frequent, which have stabilized in the form of acquired morphology. In this case, we are talking about the so-called obliterating bronchiolitis and organizing pneumonia (262, 263). At this stage, the passive attitude to the restoration of bronchial patency in patients with viral forms of AP and the strengthening of the role of hormone therapy in their treatment as a "means of salvation" contribute to an increase in such morphological consequences (201,202,204,205,365,366). Such morphological transformation after coronavirus infection is no longer uncommon in the description of the observed results, and today's recommendations for increasing the dose of corticosteroids may contribute to this.

4.2.7. Involvement of the pleural cavity in the process

In recent years, the occurrence of parapneumonic pleurisy in AP has become considered a familiar sign, the frequency of which continues to grow, reaching almost 40-60% among hospitalized patients (243-246). Unfortunately, the existing ideas about the causes of pleurisy in patients with AP were formed on the basis of the leading role of pleural infection and do not agree with the actual materials that are published on this topic.

The existing understanding of the causes and mechanisms of pleural effusion development in AP is manifested in the features of some classifications of this complication. Thus, some authors attribute parapneumonic pleurisy to primary, in contrast to secondary pleural complications arising after operations, injuries or purulent diseases of other organs (265, 266). However, the primacy of any process means the independence of its development, and not the result of the consequence of another pathology, right? The very term "parapneumonic" means that this form of pleurisy accompanies pneumonia, and does not manifest itself as an independent phenomenon.

The very fact of the appearance of pleural effusion in patients with AP is another circumstance that goes beyond the normal physiology of the lungs. External pressure on the lung tissue by the contents of the pleura and an increase in intra-thoracic pressure are inevitable pathophysiological mechanisms accompanying the appearance of pleurisy, isn't it? However, the negative effect of pleural effusion on the work of the pulmonary-cardiac apparatus does not always receive a pathogenetic assessment. Many clinicians prefer not to rush with the evacuation of exudate, especially if they assume its non-purulent nature. In such situations, well-learned principles of antibacterial therapy are manifested, according to which etiotropic drugs can solve all problems.

For example, some experts believe that pleural effusion should gradually resolve against the background of antibacterial therapy (266). The choice of such a wait-and-see tactic clearly shows that the pathogen, as the main root of the whole problem, and the belief in the universality of antibiotics dominate in modern professional ideas over the understanding of the pathogenesis of the disease and its complications. The hope for the effect of etiotropic drugs clearly exceeds the understanding of the importance of evacuation of effusion and elimination of its negative role. Or, for example, how can one explain the claim that antibiotics contribute to the disappearance of giant lung cysts after necrotic pneumonia (267)? However, in this case, these drugs are actually credited with the ability to eliminate the morphological consequences of the inflammatory process, which they initially do not possess.

Although the probability of developing pleural empyema is known already at the earliest stages of the disease, and the diagnosed pleurisy may turn out to be purulent at the first examination (245), some experts believe that there is a gradual transition from uninfected fluid to typical suppuration in the pleura (246, 268). Such reports once again raise the question of the adequacy of treatment, against which there is a further deterioration of pleural changes. In this regard, attention has already been drawn to the fact that if there is progress in the development of the disease against the background of treatment, then such treatment does not correspond to the current process.

According to the materials published by some experts, the time of development of purulent accumulation in the pleura from the first signs of the disease to the diagnosis of pleural empyema is on average 2 weeks (269, 270). At the same time, attention is drawn to the fact that in many patients with AP, signs of the disease are eliminated during this time, but in some of them the process continues to progress, despite the success of etiotropic treatment, and reaches the stage of severe complications. Paradoxical, at first glance, the nature of these data actually hides the regularity of the complicated course of AP, depending on the degree of manifestation of SIRS and the intensity of such type of medical care as infusion therapy.

In this regard, the question of modern principles of medical care and the impact of such treatment on the dynamics of inflammatory changes in lung tissue once again arises. The routine explanation of such observations by the presence of virulent pathogens does not correspond to the essence of the facts indicating the successful suppression of the infectious factor. For example, how to explain the reason for the development of pleural empyema only by its infection, if the pathogen is not detected in the purulent contents in almost half of such observations? (266, 270, 271)

In connection with the latest information, it is necessary to pay attention to such an important circumstance that, unlike the initial stages of the disease, the development of pleural empyema provides a unique opportunity to conduct a microbiological study of the material directly from the inflammation zone. In this case, there is no need to assess the questionable reliability of indirect determinations of the pathogen, such as, for example, testing of the antigen in urine. At the same time, as is known, purulent exudate is an accumulation of cells, proteins and other substances that leave tissue structures as a result of inflammatory transformations in combination with an infectious factor involved in this process.

Negative results of microbiological studies of purulent exudate from the pleura indicate the effectiveness of the use of antibiotics, but at the same time this circumstance suggests that this type of treatment does not affect the mechanisms of current inflammatory transformations. Therefore, in order to understand the causes of the progressive course of the inflammatory process after neutralization of the pathogen, the search for an answer to this question should be conducted in a different direction.

It was noted above that for the analysis of the mechanisms accompanying the development and course of AR, the most suitable model for their consideration is the variant of aggressive dynamics of the process, in which pathogenetic features are more clearly manifested. Such an analysis is necessary in order to present the entire chain of AP pathogenesis and in the future be able to purposefully apply pathogenetically based care depending on the stage of disease development.

Pathogenetic links in the dynamics of the inflammatory process in AP have their own distinctive features and characteristic manifestations that continue in a certain sequence and have a causal relationship with each other. Each stage of the disease has distinctive morphological and functional shifts that can be detected and recorded using diagnostic methods. The dilemma lies only in the angle from which the observed violations will be evaluated and interpreted, since conceptual preferences ultimately determine the entire further process of providing medical care.

For example, the rapid appearance of a pleural reaction is characteristic of aggressive forms of AP development, and the nature of the effusion reflects the features of the inflammatory process in the lung tissue. The continued accumulation of fluid in the pleural cavity is a reflection of the intensive process of exudation in the area of inflammation, and the build-up of pleurisy after the start of treatment requires, first of all, an analysis of the quality of therapy, which may include methods that can stimulate the production of exudate.

The preservation of active exudation in the area of inflammation and the insufficient effectiveness of the release of the pleural cavity from the contents create a kind of reservoir-sump. The viscosity of the exudate remaining in it begins to grow as a result of the gradual absorption of its liquid part with the concentration and precipitation of the components contained in it. As a result of such deposits, the pleural cavity begins to divide into separate chambers containing the remaining exudate.

In the case of the development of the described situation, the methods of simple removal of the contents of the pleura are already losing their capabilities and meaning, giving way to more aggressive methods of assistance. It should only be borne in mind that such states do not occur instantly. The formation of such a variant of pleural complications requires a certain amount of time, and timely adequate evacuation of exudate, which can prevent their development, is an alternative to the wait-and-see tactics often used when pleural accumulations appear.

The presented possibility of a wait-and-see tactic against the background of antibiotic treatment contradicts the opinion of other specialists who rightly believe that pleural puncture is mandatory for the primary diagnosis of pleurisy, since according to clinical data it is impossible to distinguish serous effusion from purulent (244,270). If the tactical options for solving the fate of pleural effusion may have fundamental differences, then the etiotropic treatment of PE is still unanimously recognized as the main one.

In the latter connection, it is worth noting that an overestimated assessment of the role of antibiotics in the treatment of PE cannot hide the facts noted above that in most patients the average time for the formation of this complication is about 2 weeks against the background of intensive etiotropic treatment (269, 270). At the same time, there is no reason to consider antibacterial therapy ineffective, since in half of such observations pathogenic microorganisms are not detected in the contents of the pleural cavity.

In this context, it is necessary to remember that pleural effusion is a consequence of a focus of inflammation in the lung, and its production can be maintained if exudation processes are maintained and stimulated. Such pathophysiological parallels lead to the need for a critical analysis of the treatment methods used.

The experience of AP treatment presented in the literature indicates that pleurisy in this disease in general and pleural empyema, in particular, are a sign of the most aggressive or immune to initial therapy processes. The involvement of the pleural cavity in the inflammatory process is essentially a continuation of the latter, therefore, the nature of the pleural reaction serves as a mirror image of the pathological disorders that occur in the lesion. The causal chain of these processes indicates that the successful treatment of pleurisy in AP is interrelated. first of all, with pathogenetic effects on the pulmonary focus and parallel early removal of pleural exudate.

Considering pleural complications of AP, it is impossible to ignore those of their variants that are caused by the immediate consequences of necrotic tissue damage as a result of inflammation. If the focus of necrosis is located in the cortical layers of the organ, its rejection usually occurs in the direction of the pleural cavity. Such rejections are the cause of the sudden development of pyopneumothorax, and the size of the rejection zone and the level of exposure of bronchial branches determine the presence and size of bronchopleural fistulas and other nuances of this complication. The presence of a valve mechanism in the bronchial branches open in the direction of the pleural cavity causes the development of intra-thoracic tension syndrome and requires immediate help to eliminate such a compartment syndrome.

If there is a fairly complete consensus on the cause of the development of pyopneumothorax, then the origins of mediastinal complications in bronchopulmonary inflammatory processes either in most cases remain without comment, or sometimes receive explanations that are fantastic from the point of view of anatomy. In this perspective, we are talking about complications such as pneumomediastinum and, less often, pneumopericardium. During the SARS-CoV-2 pandemic, publications about the appearance of air in the mediastinal zone began to appear more and more often, which became more frequent among those hospitalized with this infection (286-291). This requires a more detailed understanding of the mechanism of this complication in order to understand the principle of providing assistance in case of negative dynamics and signs of tension.

Pneumomediastinum and pneumopericardium are relatively rare complications that occur in various diseases of the respiratory system and can significantly worsen the condition of patients. Pneumomediastinum is observed in literary representations much more often than pneumopericardium, but the mechanism of their occurrence, from my point of view, is identical, therefore it is better to focus on the ways of the appearance of air in the mediastinal fiber when there are more options for its penetration compared to the cardiac bag.

This complication occurs not only in patients with inflammatory lung diseases, but even in conditions that are not directly related to this system, for example, in women in labor (292). This fact suggests that an important triggering factor of this phenomenon is sudden attacks of increased intrabronchial pressure. Such a sudden increase in air pressure in a confined space, according to Pascal's law (293), spreads evenly in all directions and can create a flow of air to the surrounding tissues, creating defects in the weakest or damaged tissues.

Free air in the mediastinum can appear from anatomical spaces that have a connection with it, which corresponds to the anatomy of the body and physical laws. For example, even in patients with COVID-19 pneumonia, it is logical to look for esophageal damage as the cause of pneumomediastinum and perform esophagography if there are relevant suspicions (294). However, a number of authors describe the mechanism of development of such complications as a result of damage to the alveolar parts of the lung, considering that air enters the mediastinal tissue through perivascular spaces (295-298). This mechanism of involvement in the mediastinal process in inflammatory diseases of the respiratory system seems unrealistic in the light of existing circumstances and facts.

First of all, there is no objective evidence that air enters the mediastinum through the perivascular spaces as a result of damage to tissue barriers in the alveolar parts of the lungs. This path of air propagation should not only be visible, but also very clearly distinguishable on X-rays and, especially, on tomograms. Before entering the mediastinum, the air must create accumulations around the vessels with significant tissue stratification. It can't enter the mediastinum through the perivascular spaces without leaving any traces in them, right? In addition, the mediastinum is the next stage of air propagation and should contain less of it than the tissues from which it comes. This is simple physics, and the predominance of air in the mediastinum over its volume in the lung tissue can only be in the presence of a valve mechanism. However, the presence of free air at the site of tissue damage should be constant, regardless of the further conditions of its spread.

The mechanism of air leakage from the parenchymal parts of the lungs has no confirmation in the results of visual diagnostics. If you look at the illustrations given in the articles on this topic noted above, then not only on simple radiographs, but even on tomograms of lungs with a large amount of air in the mediastinum, there are no hints of its presence in the perivascular tissues of the organ itself.

In fact, the localization of the cause of pneumomediastinum has a purely anatomical explanation. The mediastinal cavity surrounds most of the trachea and the proximal sections of the main bronchi, slightly deepening in the area of the gate in the direction of the lung, but has no other anatomical connections with the structures located inside the organ. Therefore, tissue defects in the form of small cracks through which air enters the mediastinum can be located in the initial sections of the main bronchi or in the trachea. In this regard, attention should be paid to anatomical postmortem examinations for coronavirus infection, which showed the presence of small foci of necrosis in the wall of the trachea and the main bronchi (285). In addition, pneumomediastinum in most patients, whose materials are given in the literature, arose against the background of positive pressure ventilation.

An accurate lifetime diagnosis of such microcracks in the initial sections of the tracheobronchial tree remains, as a rule, unrealized, but confirmation of this source of air leakage into the surrounding tissues can be easily obtained with a postmortem examination of the tightness of the respiratory tract. To do this, during the autopsy, the pulmonary complex is immersed under water and air is injected into it through a cannula or endotracheal tube using a breathing nozzle. The area of the defect can be easily detected by the release of air bubbles and further subject this area to a more detailed examination, including histological examination. This technique was used by the author of these lines for postmortem diagnosis of the source of pneumomediastinum in previous years and can be easily reproduced at the present time as an objective confirmation of the origin of the complication.

The need to clarify the mechanism of occurrence of pneumomediastinum is of great practical importance, since in the case of intra-thoracic compression syndrome, patients need immediate help. Understanding the origins and essence of this complication allows you to purposefully apply the most effective methods of medical care without wasting time on additional diagnostics, the methods of which in clinical situations with this complication usually do not give decisive results.

Pneumopericardium in inflammatory processes of the respiratory system is observed much less frequently than pneumomediastinum, although during the SARS-CoV-2 pandemic, observations of such complications began to occur more frequently (288,299-303). The occurrence of pneumomediastinum hypothetically seems to many authors to be more easily explained, compared with pneumopericardium. This deceptive impression is formed as a result of the fact that the air that has penetrated into the mediastinum is able to freely spread further, manifesting itself as subcutaneous emphysema in the neck, face, upper chest. The latter sign is due to the fact that the mediastinal cavity has its continuation without anatomical obstacles in two directions - to the neck and to the retroperitoneal space.

The development of an isolated pneumopericardium from the point of view of anatomy as a whole at first glance seems to be a fantastic phenomenon, since the cardiac chemise is a closed anatomical formation that has no options for air penetration, and in clinical observations of the complication that has arisen, this is confirmed by the absence of its further spread from the pericardium. However, the known anatomical features do not prevent different authors from considering the unlikely mechanisms of this complication in conditions of respiratory diseases.

The standard explanation of the mechanism of the pneumopericardium is a scheme similar to the development of pneumomediastinum: damage to the alveolar parts of the lung with the spread of air through the perivasal and peribronchial tissues (299-301). Probably, realizing the doubtfulness of such air penetration into the pericardium, some experts suggest additional mechanisms. So, after the appearance of air in the mediastinum, A. Singh et al. (302) a stratification of the paraaortic tissue with the formation of a pathway to the pericardium is suspected, and H. Zhu and J.J. Lieber (303) hypothesize inflammatory damage to the pericardial wall. And again, as in explaining the causes of pneumomediastinum, no one pays attention to the absence of signs of free air during its intended progress, which is demonstrated by the illustrations given, especially indicative of an isolated pneumopericardium.

By the way, the pneumopericardium, which is considered as a pathology requiring differential diagnosis with pneumomediastinum (295), has an identical mechanism of development. The source of free air in the pericardium is a microtrauma of the tracheal bifurcation area and the initial sections of the main bronchi, which are anatomically partially located in the cavity of the cardiac shirt. This anatomical feature is used in thoracic surgery to perform transpericardial interventions on these areas of the tracheobronchial tree. The source of this complication can also be identified and investigated, but only with the help of the postmortem method described above. Unfortunately, methods of simple lifetime diagnosis of such causes have not yet been developed.

4.3. Requirements for the disease doctrine

The idea of the essence of AP should be based on the general biological and medical canons of science. The lack of due attention to these fundamental principles can form a distortion of views on the causes and consequences of the occurrence and development of the disease. In order to understand what canons of science we are talking about, it is necessary to evaluate once again how fully and comprehensively the classics of the inflammatory process and the peculiarities of the individual reaction of the body to this phenomenon are presented in the modern concept of AP. Such an analysis shows that the modern ideas about this disease require a thorough and detailed restoration of the role and significance of many factors of these phenomena.

An important place in the process of forming such a worldview should also be occupied by the functions inherent in the affected organ, the violation of which inevitably accompanies its inflammation and determines the features and uniqueness of the disease. How successfully can the discussed problem be solved today if the place and importance of the lungs in the circulatory system, their unique parameters of blood flow and their role in regulating the entire system are well known, but these features are not given importance in the process of diagnosis and therapeutic correction? In this case, there can be only one answer, but so far the results of modern views on the essence of the problem reflect the indicators of current statistics.

It is very important to have an idea not only about the clinical manifestation of individual links of the pathological process and their interpretation based on the results of modern diagnostic tests and procedures, but also about their significance in the overall system of adaptation of the body to new unexpected conditions. In this regard, it is necessary to continue clarifying the permissible criteria for such deviations that correspond to the terms "adaptation", "compensation", "norm in pathology". Such studies should allow us to differentially determine the choice of therapeutic measures from a new point of view, replacing the stereotypes of medical care, which are currently a mandatory "therapeutic stamp" regardless of the clinical features and stage of the disease.

The main section in the AP doctrine is the description of the pathogenesis of the disease, which should reflect the sequence and stages of the development of the process. Such a chain of mechanisms corresponding to the increasing manifestations of the disease serves as a guideline for determining and selecting the necessary means of assistance, as well as for determining the limits of the effectiveness of individual techniques and the limits of the reversibility of the process. This is especially important in conditions of rapid dynamics of the process, when timely emergency and targeted assistance is needed.

All these remarks about the principles of bringing the AP doctrine in line with the fundamentals of medical science belong to the fundamental section in solving the problem under discussion, since the current concept of this independent nosology has no fundamental differences from other inflammatory processes. The general scheme of the development of inflammatory diseases, regardless of the localization of their primary focus, has the characteristics of the pathogen as the main criterion, which, when assessing the condition of patients with AP, depersonalizes the exceptional features of this disease. Evaluation on the same scale of multidirectional circulatory disorders led, from my point of view, to overdiagnosis of septic complications of AP and a shift in therapeutic efforts.

The long overdue need for a radical revision of views on the nature of acute inflammation of the lung tissue is confirmed by another non-standard information. In previous years, in private conversations, I had to hear from interlocutors who did not have a medical education, very sharp, but reasoned remarks about the effectiveness of modern healthcare systems. Today, this topic has not only reached the level of a broad and open discussion. A little more than 10 years ago, a proposal was put forward in China to create a so-called integrative medicine, the idea of which originated (!) in the Academy of Engineering (210). The purpose of this proposal is to involve in solving medical problems not only professional specialists of medical professions, but also representatives of a wide range of other sciences (biology, chemistry, physics, economics, psychology, law, management, ecology, etc.).

Integrative medicine was developed in order to help modern official medicine at the state level. Today, the first results of such work are already being offered for review to the international community as confirmation of successful cooperation of specialists of various profiles in the field of healthcare (211). However, in this context, attention is attracted not by a new form of cooperation between scientists, but by the reasons for its occurrence. It seems that the faith in the reliability of healthcare systems among potential patients has been significantly shaken, and their most active group is trying to use non-medical experience and knowledge to improve medical research and services.

The latter assumptions receive very serious confirmation if we quote a small quote from the above-mentioned article (211). The author of the article, Jun M., who, according to the accompanying information, is not a doctor, writes the following:

> *"The main problems in the clinical medical research on the prevention and management of NCP (Novel Coronavirus Pneumonia) in China the main features of the clinical medical research on the prevention and management of NCP in China are as follows: These microscopic results cannot reflect the overall characteristics of the human body, the human body specimens to be transferred outside the body to explore, so that in vitro discovery cannot fully explain the situation inside the body; Conclusions drawn from the human anatomy sometimes do not really describe the functional characteristics of the human body and so on [1(210)]. These clinical studies are of little significance to the clinical work of*

the prevention, treatment and health management of NCP. Advances in clinical research in the prevention, treatment and management of NCP should serve human health rather than focusing on publication, citation, and number of influencing factors. However, many clinical research papers on the prevention, treatment and management of NCP do not really contribute to human health."

The level and capabilities of modern official medicine in China do not differ much from health systems in other developed countries, so such an unflattering characteristic of this industry may cause objections from many of its representatives. However, before protesting, it makes sense to carefully weigh and evaluate the actual situation in this section. In the end, it is precisely these aspects of the problem, only in a less harsh and less categorical presentation, that this book is devoted to. The reason for writing it, as already noted above, was the distortion of views on the nature of AP, the tendency to increase virtual representations of the disease at the cellular and molecular levels, the loss of specific features of the pulmonary localization of the process and its evaluation in clinical settings according to a template with other variants of inflammation.

In order to more fully characterize the current situation in the area of the problem under discussion, it is necessary to look at this situation from the opposite side of the globe from China. In this case, we are talking about approaches to solving this problem in the United States, where the level of medicine and scientific research is deservedly considered one of the highest in the world.

So, as of January 2021, the National Institutes of Health (NIH) in the United States issued almost a thousand awards totaling about $ 2 billion to support research projects on COVID-19, but the results of the overwhelming number of such works remain unknown (304). Only the materials of 8% of completed or discontinued (!?) works were published in the database, which operates under the auspices of the US National Library of Medicine (ClinicalTrials.gov). This database contains the results of private and publicly funded clinical trials conducted worldwide. These statistics clearly show how low the return on medical science funding is in a society that traditionally knows how to manage its money.

The presented materials look even more depressing if we take into account the fact that the United States confidently leads the world throughout the SARS-CoV-2 pandemic not only in the number of infected, but also in the number of deaths from COVID-19 pneumonia (305). The similarity of statistical indicators among those infected with coronavirus, who have a very virulent pathogen and who are deprived of direct etiotropic treatment, and CAP patients who have a choice of etiotropic drugs has already been discussed above. However, by analogy with previous ideas about inflammatory processes of the lungs, the American health care system, like all world medicine, is making titanic efforts to find means to counteract the causative agent of the current pandemic, ignoring the need for a radical revision of the strategy for solving the problem of AP.

All these results, from my point of view, are quite logical and are due to the prevailing ideology of the AP. However, contrary to logic and professional analysis of severe inflammatory processes of lung tissue, the search for answers to questions sometimes takes an unexpected direction. For example, one of the leading and most authoritative journals in the medical world, *The New England Journal of Medicine*, in its editorial directly examines the cause of the widespread spread of coronavirus in American society and the subsequent increase in mortality rates during the pandemic as a result of incorrect government decisions (306).

The spread of coronavirus can be considered as a phenomenon that depends on epidemiological decisions at the state level only to a certain extent and with reservations, since within the framework of the current pandemic it became obvious that the introduction of strict isolation in a number of countries could not fully protect their populations from the next waves of infection. At the same time, the direction and validity of medical efforts to treat hospitalized patients can in no way be attributed to the country's leadership, especially since the health care system enjoys full support and provision from the state in accordance with its own requests. Therefore, the causes of high mortality should be sought in another direction, and since this path actually depends entirely on the quality of medical care, it may be advisable to conduct a detailed analysis of this section?

The latest example of the opinion of well-known experts on the existing problem is another indication of how much the role of the pathogen dominates the ideas about the problem of AP. During the SARS-CoV-2 pandemic, it has already become obvious that not all those infected with coronavirus need additional medical care and, moreover, hospitalization. Epidemiological statistics give an idea of the speed and extent of the spread of coronavirus, but not about the results and consequences of such contact. In addition, it is well known that the epidemiological situation depends not only on the introduction of social and other preventive measures, but also on the understanding of the situation, responsibility and consciousness of each citizen.

While representatives of medicine see the fault of the state administration in indecisive and insufficiently stringent social measures to reduce contacts in society during the pandemic (306), judicial authorities consider complaints from population groups in which the latter, on the contrary, consider such measures infringing on their civil rights (307). Regardless of how such social clashes are regarded, the statistics of the pandemic in different countries show that it is impossible to identify a direct relationship between the degree of spread of the coronavirus and the number of patients requiring hospitalization, as well as the number of deaths. These statistics do not depend on the socio-economic situation of different countries. Moreover, the leaders with the highest relative mortality from COVID-19 pneumonia include the most developed countries (305).

In the latter connection, the significance of medical claims against the state administration, from my point of view, has a completely different intuitive and hidden meaning. The problem that the pandemic has revealed today has existed for many years and is not the number of infected people, but the quality of medical care for hospitalized people. And it is at this crucial stage, when fast and effective specialized care is required, the latter, despite the dedication of the medical staff of numerous hospitals around the world, is of an auxiliary and palliative nature. The results of such assistance are quite expected.

The importance of the causative agent as the main cause of AP continues to dominate the ideology of the disease, but now this thesis has become overgrown with fear and uncertainty, since the emergence of a new pathogen has deprived medicine of its main trump card - etiotropic treatment. Plans to get out of this situation continue to be formed on the basis of the idea of suppressing the infectious onset, but while everyone is waiting for another miracle and hoping to find an effective antiviral agent, patients with coronavirus pneumonia continue to be admitted to hospitals, whose clinic reflects not indicative signs of a viral infection, but a picture of a violent reaction of the body to the inflammatory process in the lung.

The dominant AP concept is a powerful obstacle in solving this problem. In recent years, the importance of the pathogen as the main and only cause of the disease has actually become an axiom, limiting the direction of research on this problem and narrowing the choice of therapeutic agents. Without a revision of these guidelines, which do not take into account the classical canons of medical and biological science, the successful solution of the problem of AP will remain an open question.

4.4. The main provisions of the doctrine of acute pneumonia

1. AP is a classic example of acute inflammation. The main and characteristic feature of this disease is the inflammatory process, which throughout the foreseeable history has determined its terminology and place in the classification of nosological forms. Acute inflammation of the lung tissue has clinical, laboratory and pathomorphological criteria, of which the latter criterion is the most important. The pathological transformation of the lung tissue creates conditions for the detection of this area with the help of radiation diagnostics. The classical recognition of this disease consists precisely in the detection of inflammatory changes in the organ tissue, which, in combination with certain clinical and laboratory abnormalities, indicate the localization and nature of the process.

2. AP belongs to the category of acute inflammatory processes of nonspecific etiology. The absence of one specific pathogen, which is an inseparable root cause of AP, serves as an important distinguishing feature of this disease. The list of AP pathogens, among which bacteria and viruses predominate, is quite extensive, and the leaders of this list periodically and unpredictably change, but the main signs and criteria of the disease remain unchanged.

3. Pathogenic microorganisms are one of the provoking factors of inflammation in the lung tissue, but not the main and only cause of the disease. Possible pathogens of AP are mainly representatives of the symbiotic microflora of the body, and even the presence of the most virulent and antibiotic-resistant strains among them does not mean the threat of mandatory development of AP (61-63). Such agents can endlessly get along with the body, but then they can cause diseases under certain conditions and in combination with other stimuli. Even the transmission of an atypical infectious agent with a high potential for the development of inflammation in the lungs from a sick person to a healthy person is not an absolute

condition for the development of AP, which is clearly demonstrated by the statistics of viral epidemics and the SARS-CoV-2 pandemic (17-20).

4. The body's reaction to the effects of both infectious and non-infectious stimuli is manifested by a set of signs that are currently defined as SIRS. This syndrome, which replaced the old concept of reactivity, characterizes the body's ability to respond to various stimuli, and the scenario for the development of such a syndrome is the same, since it reflects the overall reaction of the body. The range of such reactions is endless - from barely noticeable to overly aggressive and is a purely individual characteristic that determines the difference in the clinical picture of one disease.

5. In addition to the individual characteristics of the general reaction of the body, the specificity of clinical manifestations of acute inflammation depends on the localization of the primary focus and dysfunction of the affected organ, since the inflammatory process is inevitably accompanied by five classic signs, among which dysfunction determines the characteristics of a particular disease.

6. Among all known acute inflammatory processes, AP is the only nosology that is localized in the area of the small circle of blood circulation. The fundamental differences between the functional purpose and the parameters of the small and large circulatory circles are the cause of various mechanisms of peripheral circulatory disorders. Disorders of systemic blood flow in AP are secondary in nature, indirectly reflecting the catastrophe of pulmonary circulation and the desire of the body to maintain parity in the circulatory system. Such a mechanism of circulatory disorders is inherent only in this nosological form and is fundamentally different from similar shifts accompanying other localization of inflammation.

7. The sequence of systemic circulatory disorders in AP leads in the most severe situations to the development of a typical picture of shock, but the reasons for its special origin require a separate designation of this variant of shock as pulmonogenic. The possibility

of generalization of infection in patients with AP exists, as with any inflammatory disease of non-specific etiology, but the development of this complication may be a layering on already existing homeostasis shifts inherent in this pathology, and the fact of the occurrence of such complications requires objective confirmation, and not assumptions based on analogies and indirect signs.

8. The basis of the inflammatory transformation of lung tissue in AP is a classical vascular reaction with a certain change in the stages of this process, which is accompanied by a sharp increase in the permeability of the vascular wall and pathological movement of intravascular components into the extravascular space. In the case of aggressive development of an inflammatory reaction, a rapid increase in the volume of tissues in this zone exerts external pressure on the vessels and changes their architectonics. As a result, there is a shift in the proportions between the arterial and venous sectors towards the predominance of blood delivery over its outflow, up to a complete stop of blood flow, disruption of tissue nutrition and their subsequent necrosis.

9. Bronchial vessels, which have significantly higher blood pressure compared to the pulmonary network and have shunting messages with the latter, can affect excessive blood filling of inflamed areas of the organ, contributing to total necrosis of the lobe. This postulate needs further study.

10. The blockade of bronchial branches in the area of inflammation not only complements the reasons for the cessation of ventilation of the corresponding alveolar sections, but also disrupts their natural drainage, preventing the recovery processes. The most effective of the natural defense mechanisms for recanalization of the bronchial tract is cough.

11. Exudation in the focus of inflammation, exceeding the drainage capabilities of pleural reabsorption mechanisms, contributes to the accumulation of excess tissue fluid in the pleural cavity. This fluid is a consequence of the inflammatory process in the lung tissue, so it

borrows its signs and repeats the characteristics of the severity of the organ lesion. The intensity of exudative processes increases in parallel with the activity of the inflammatory process, and the development of pleurisy is always secondary to AP.

12. The appearance of air in the pleural cavity is the result of emptying necrotic areas of lung tissue into it, while air entering the mediastinum or pericardium occurs due to small areas of necrosis and microcracks in the bifurcation of the trachea and proximal sections of the main bronchi. The latter circumstance indicates that endobronchial inflammation in patients with AP accompanies the disease much more often than it is diagnosed and taken into account in treatment.

4.5. A brief interpretation of the doctrine of acute pneumonia

A few decades ago, the vast majority of cases of AP occurred with the participation of bacteria, which to one degree or another were symbionts of the organism. Despite the long-term advantage of pneumococcus in this process, no direct infections with this pathogen were observed, and its frequent presence among the accompanying microorganisms allowed the body to maintain parity. Additional factors and conditions were required for the occurrence of inflammation in the lung tissue. Most often, viral and colds created the ground for this.

The discovery of antibiotics and the beginning of their widespread clinical use gradually changed the usual relationship between the body and its microflora. Purposeful suppression of some types of pathogens began to manifest itself by strengthening the role of others. Antibiotic-resistant strains have appeared, which are increasingly being detected in healthy people. Finally, in recent decades, there has been a gradual but steady increase in the viral etiology of pneumonia, which is a consequence of prolonged "sterilizing" therapy of this disease.

In recent years, inflammatory lung diseases of viral etiology (mainly influenza) have usually been the result of seasonal epidemics, which gave reason to consider these pathogens a non-standard infection from the outside and prompted the annual vaccination of the population. Nevertheless, during the periods of traditional influenza epidemics and the current SARS-CoV-2 pandemic, a huge number of people around the globe tolerate such contacts easily and unnoticeably, even without prior vaccination. For the occurrence of an inflammatory process in the lung tissue, additional conditions are necessary in the form of aggravating factors that unite patients into so-called risk groups. In addition, the growing allergization of the population, air pollution and certain atmospheric conditions contribute to the occurrence of the disease.

Under the influence of various internal and external factors that reduce the protective mechanisms, contacts of the structures of the respiratory system with substances to which the body is hypersensitive and reacts with an immune response are especially dangerous. Such a reaction creates a place of initial tissue damage with an increase in their vulnerability to representatives of the microflora penetrating into these departments. With such a bronchogenic beginning of the process, one of the inevitable manifestations is endobronchitis with a violation of the drainage functions of the corresponding branches. Narrowing of the bronchial lumen leads to a decrease in ventilation and a change in blood flow in the corresponding parts of the parenchyma. Once in the zone of such changes, potential pathogens no longer meet proper resistance and receive conditions favorable for their aggressive behavior.

It is known that at the cellular and molecular level there are differences between bacterial and viral forms of the inflammatory process. For example, in order for viral inflammation to begin, the pathogen must not just be in this zone, but penetrate into the cell. Today, during the SARS-CoV-2 pandemic, the theory of creating barriers to the penetration of coronavirus into the cell has become especially relevant and the number of publications with such proposals is constantly growing, forming the impression that a breakthrough on this front will help patients with viral pneumonia. However, do not be mistaken about this, living in anticipation of the next panacea. If these expectations can be realized, they are unlikely to be able to seriously help those who are already ill.

If effective means are created against the intracellular penetration of viruses, then this will undoubtedly be a big step towards the prevention of viral diseases, but not their treatment. In this case, the situation is discussed when the virus has already penetrated the cell and the inflammatory process is a fait accompli. In these conditions, it is necessary to look for another goal for the direction of therapeutic actions in order to get the desired result. In order not to create another mirage in search of effective remedies for an existing disease, it is necessary to pay attention to one very significant feature of the current reality.

Information on this topic testifies to the undoubted fact that, despite the noticeable differences between bacterial and viral inflammation at the molecular and cellular levels, it is not possible to carry out a clear differential diagnosis between these forms of the disease at the level of clinical symptoms. The absence of clinical cardinal differences between inflammatory processes of the lungs of different etiologies is quite a logical and natural consequence of morphofunctional changes in the organ. The independence of the clinical picture of AP from its etiology clearly indicates the leading role of the focus of inflammation in the formation of the main signs of the disease. Insufficient attention to this obvious fact will remain a serious obstacle to solving the AP problem.

Attempts at differential diagnosis of AP on etiological grounds are one of the reflections of the current trend in the study of this problem with the search for solutions at the cellular and molecular level. The predominance of such aspirations in clinical situations has led to the emergence of new organizational approaches in the form of so-called integrative medicine. This form of cooperation between researchers in various fields of science can certainly bring tangible results, but an effective solution to the problem of AP will still depend on professional medical views on the causes and consequences underlying it. In this regard, the above quote about the reasons for the birth of integrative medicine accurately reflects the difficulties that have accumulated in clinical disciplines (211).

Elucidation of the etiology of AP is currently subordinated only to solving the question of the need for the use of antibiotics, which, as the years of recent decades show, have also failed to successfully solve the problem under discussion. In a real situation, the pathogen does not determine the clinic of the disease and the severity of the patients' condition. Those signs that are formed under the influence of the focus of inflammation, regardless of which pathogen causes this process, require other therapeutic approaches. Therefore, when therapeutic efforts are focused on suppressing the pathogen, the body must independently correct deviations in the work of its main systems. How successful such a correction is can be traced by the statistical dynamics of the results.

One of the initial mechanisms of inflammation that trigger the chain of pathological transformation of tissues is arterial hyperemia in the area of injury, when the body tries to deliver the maximum possible amount of cellular and humoral protective factors to this area by increasing blood flow. This circumstance is a protective reaction to the damage that has occurred, and this mechanism works autonomously. The positive orientation of this mechanism is obvious, but it causes new deviations in the usual constants of the body, which, in turn, require an additional reaction.

An increase in blood flow to one of the departments of the small circulatory circle is accompanied by an increase in pressure in these vessels and the appearance of signals from their baroreceptors. At this stage of the development of the process, clinical symptoms will depend on the rate of current changes in the focus of inflammation and the corresponding rate of further deviations. In fact, in this situation we are talking about an individual reaction of the body to damage to its structure, which is now commonly called SIRS. This reaction is one of the individual characteristics of our body, and there can be as many variants of such a reaction as fingerprints. The variant of this answer determines the clinical manifestation of AP, which may differ significantly in different patients. The essence of emerging adaptive mechanisms can be presented in two diametrically opposite situations.

In a situation where the inflammatory process in the lung is characterized by a relatively slow development, blood flow to the affected area and an increase in pressure in the pulmonary vessels will also not differ in speed. The gradual strengthening of signals from the baroreceptors of the inflammatory zone prompts the body to begin the process of gradual deposition of circulating blood. With such a "leisurely" variant of development, the adaptation of the cardiovascular system to new conditions can proceed without external signs. In such cases, the body has enough time to deposit some of the circulating blood and reduce its flow to the lungs, so systemic blood pressure can remain stable.

Even a gradual decrease in the volume of circulating blood inevitably reduces peripheral microcirculation and worsens the supply of body tissues. The manifestation of these changes in the circulatory system in patients with AP can be considered such common signs as pallor, malaise, fatigue, drowsiness, decreased appetite.

Another extreme variant of SIRS is the rapid development of the inflammatory process, the speed of which leaves the body no time for gradual and easy adaptation. Rapid blood filling of the lung tissue in the affected area leads to a rapid increase in blood pressure in the pulmonary vessels, which is the reason for the fastest possible response. Irritation of baroreceptors in the inflammatory zone is accompanied by reflex connection to the reaction of the entire small circle basin, which reacts with generalized spasm of small vessels, as well as reflex hypotension of the vessels of the large circle (discharge reflex).

As a result of these protective mechanisms, the body manages to somewhat reduce the risk of the spread of inflammatory pulmonary edema, but these autonomous reactions generate the automatic launch of new reactions. Spasm of small vessels of the small circle reduces the efficiency of alveolar gas exchange, and the development of hypoxemia stimulates an increase in respiratory excursions. An increase in the respiratory rate has a massaging effect on the lung tissue, which implies a relief of blood flow through the spasmodic vessels of the small circle, although this mechanism is probably able to increase the volume of blood passing through it. As this fragment of the AP pathogenesis shows, protective and adaptive mechanisms at a certain stage of development can acquire an uncontrolled character and lead to the emergence of a vicious circle.

Reflex reduction of systemic arterial pressure allows for a short period of time to keep part of the circulating blood in it and thereby reduce venous return. In the most aggressive cases of AP development, such a change in peripheral blood flow is manifested by a clinical picture of shock. The peculiarity of this mechanism is most clearly manifested in pulmonary embolism, when a sudden reflex from the baroreceptors can be accompanied by an equally unexpected collapse. In AP, unlike thromboembolism, the manifestation of the reflex mechanism does not occur so quickly, so the body reacts to a drop in systemic blood pressure in the form of activation of humoral factors to maintain peripheral vascular tone and, in particular, the excitation of the renin-angiotensin-aldosterone system.

In the latter case, another vicious circle is clearly visible, resulting from the automatic connection of adaptive mechanisms. Even such a generalized idea of the sequence and interdependence of adaptive reactions makes it possible to understand the place and significance of generally accepted methods for assessing hemodynamic disorders in patients with AP and the expected effect of medical care if it is aimed at correcting mainly the results of final reactions in the general chain.

The brief interpretation of the AP doctrine presented above contains only the most important fragment of this information, which gives an idea of the causes of the severe course of this disease and has a direct connection with the features of diagnosis and the choice of emergency care. The nuances of local tissue transformation in the focus of inflammation do not have such a significant impact on the overall clinical picture and the choice of treatment method. They were discussed in sufficient detail above. In addition, the description of the details of the process at the cellular and molecular level does not play a strategic role in solving clinical problems.

In the latter connection, it is probably necessary to pay attention once again to the peculiarities of changes in angioarchitectonics in the area of inflammation, which develop as a result of increased permeability of the vascular wall with an increase in edema and infiltration of tissues. Changing the proportions in throughput between the arterial and venous sectors creates a kind of "vascular trap" mechanism that should be taken into account when conducting medical procedures. Under these conditions, the use of methods that can increase blood flow to the area of inflammation can stimulate further edema and infiltration of tissues, accelerating the onset of the stage of blood flow blockade and subsequent necrosis.

In general, the presented brief interpretation of the AP doctrine can serve as a direct guide for practical application. This statement is based on the personal experience of the author, who successfully used this scheme of AP pathogenesis to choose treatment methods depending on the manifestations of the disease. Currently, in the light of the dominant worldviews on this problem, it will be difficult to imagine and avoid a skeptical assessment of the fact that more than 30 years ago the author stopped considering antibiotics as the leading, and even more so the only method of treating AP. Nevertheless, the results achieved were the best confirmation of the correctness of this direction. Since then, the situation in this section of medicine has become more expressive and alarming, and the current results indicate the need for a serious and radical revision of the ideology of the disease.

CHAPTER 5

PRINCIPLES OF PROVIDING MEDICAL CARE FOR ACUTE PNEUMONIA

5.1. Current priorities in the treatment of patients with acute pneumonia

For many years before the outbreak of the SARS-CoV-2 pandemic, the question of where to start treating patients with AP and what is the main means of such assistance was not even on the agenda. In all manuals and monographs, as well as in major review and analytical articles on community-acquired pneumonia, the "Treatment" section traditionally began with a listing and description of the most appropriate antibiotics for this group of patients. Such a list was usually presented in the form of sequential characteristics, often summarized in large tables, and formed the main part of this item. The remaining therapeutic agents were given as additional methods.

This order of priorities was familiar, universally recognized and indisputable, and the treatment of most patients with AP was considered for a long time as "antibiotics alone". In the case of severe development of the disease with signs of septic complications, it was expected to succeed with the help of the fastest possible administration of antibiotics to such patients in order to give them the status of first and emergency care. For example, in some studies, it is recommended to use antibiotics already in the first hour of hospitalization, noting that such a measure, together with a general set of additional measures, slightly reduces mortality in sepsis (173,308,309). Other observations show that the initiation of antibacterial therapy with a difference of several hours does not significantly affect subsequent results (310,311).

The desire to give antibiotics the status of first and emergency care does not take into account one important circumstance. Antimicrobials, even in the case of rapid and maximum effectiveness, eliminate only one of the etiological factors, while the clinical symptoms and severity of the patients' condition are due to a violation of the function of the affected organ as a result of the inflammatory process. In this regard, successful sterilization of the inflammatory zone cannot instantly alleviate the condition of the patient, whose body needs additional help to slow down the process and then eliminate tissue transformation.

Even more problematic is the hope for the effect of antiviral drugs. Viruses, unlike bacteria, are already inside the cells by the time the focus of inflammation in the lung is diagnosed, and the possibility of their rapid and direct contact with drugs will be very difficult, especially if you take into account microcirculation disorders in these areas. Therefore, the hope for a radical solution to the problem of viral pneumonia in the case of the development of effective antiviral drugs is not entirely realistic.

In recent years, when the viral nature of AP was suspected, some antiviral drugs were used in addition to antibiotics (199,308,310), but in the current SARS-CoV-2 pandemic, a large number of such patients were left without conventional etiotropic therapy. No means of suppressing coronavirus comparable to the action of antibiotics have yet been found, but in this situation, illusions about the limitless possibilities of antibiotics continue to operate. Methods of verification of bacterial pathogens of AP remained the same with indirect (not from the focus of inflammation) examination of the material and questionable accuracy of the results. Bacterial coinfection using such methods is detected in a small percentage of cases (109-111), but antibiotics that do not have an antiviral effect continue to receive from 70-80% to 100% of patients with COVID-19 pneumonia (109,111-118).

Such an emergency and unreasonable variant of etiotropic therapy of viral inflammation cannot bring the expected effect, which is confirmed by numerous current publications on this section of medical care, but some specialists continue to search in vain for the optimal type of antibiotics for this group of patients (110,313,314). The loss of confidence in the traditional success of antibiotics has forced modern medicine to pay more attention to those signs of the disease that most experts consider leading - tachypnea and hypoxemia (118,312).

Some experts do not attach importance to the new etiological circumstances and recommend continuing treatment of pneumonia caused by COVID-19 with antibiotics as long as hypoxemia persists and respiratory support is required (110). The reason for the increased frequency of respiratory excursions and a decrease in blood oxygen saturation is usually explained by a violation of gas diffusion as a result of inflammatory edema of part of the alveoli (38, 174, 198), and the main attempts to get out of this impasse are aimed at increasing the concentration of oxygen in the inhaled air.

Currently, oxygen supply to patients with AP is the most common type of medical care and in most cases the first procedure that is performed to such patients. Increased interest in oxygen therapy began to manifest itself with the onset of the SARS-CoV-2 pandemic. This phenomenon can be explained by the fact that in the conditions of loss of habitual confidence in the action of etiotropic drugs, there was no simpler way in the list of therapeutic measures that would correspond to modern ideas about the mechanisms of AP development.

However, the vast experience gained when using oxygen supply during AP has shown that a simple increase in its concentration in the inhaled air does not have a fundamental effect on the condition of patients. This was the impetus for the search for such methods of oxygen supply, which, in conditions of a decrease in the area of gas exchange, could increase its concentration in the blood.

In connection with the latter, the popularity of oxygen supply to the prone positioning has returned (28,157,315-321), the technique of using a nasal cannula with a high flow (318) has been advertised. However, comparative studies of various oxygen supply methods have not revealed significant differences in their effectiveness (319,320). An even more unexpected result of the analysis of oxygen therapy was the absence of any dependence of mortality on the achieved level of blood oxygenation (321), and this absolutely clearly shows that this direction of medical care cannot help in solving the problem of AP.

Even theoretically, oxygen therapy cannot affect the causes of respiratory disorders, therefore, the further dynamics of the current inflammatory process in the most aggressive situations leads to the need for auxiliary lung ventilation or connection of extracorporeal membrane blood oxygenation (ECMO). The hope for these methods does not meet expectations, since mortality in the group of patients with AP who use these auxiliary procedures increases significantly, increasing by two or more times (29,209,322,323). In this regard, M. L. Hepokoski et al. (157) it is rightly argued that the effectiveness of ECMO in patients with AP is not proven and is very doubtful.

Another method of first aid in the hospitalization of patients over the past many decades is infusion therapy. This technique is widely used during the hospitalization of emergency patients, regardless of the nature of the disease, and if intravenous administration of antibiotics is required, patients are immediately connected to the intravenous infusion system. The crucial importance of this technique for patients with AP, especially in the early stages of the disease, has not yet been widely understood, and various proofs of its negative effect on the dynamics of inflammation in the lungs have been presented above.

Moreover, if AP is characterized by aggressive development and the patient has a decrease in peripheral blood pressure, then infusion therapy becomes a mandatory type of treatment. With such observations, experts strongly recommend injecting solutions into the venous bed in the form of boluses at the rate of 30 ml / kg for at least 3 hours (25,82, 86, 105, 125,324,325). The reasons for the ineffectiveness of this treatment in many patients and the frequent need for subsequent use of vasopressors (6.82, 105, 173), as well as the origin of pleural effusion in 40-60% of those hospitalized with AP (243-246,326), can be understood and explained on the basis of the materials presented above. Meanwhile, the negative dynamics in such patients continue to be explained solely by the influence of infection without convincing evidence of this assumption.

As the real situation shows, the most common methods of first aid in AP do not provide a guaranteed improvement in the condition of these patients. The disease, despite intensive medical efforts, continues to progress so much that critical situations that were absent at the time of hospitalization may develop already during treatment and follow-up of patients (85,158). The low effectiveness of the efforts made became much more noticeable during the SARS-CoV-2 pandemic. When patients with COVID-19 pneumonia began to concentrate in specialized departments for this purpose, the staff working in them faced the heaviest moral burden, observing the mass phenomenon of the inability of therapeutic measures to stop the development of the process (30-34).

The current situation contributed to the intensification of the search and testing of specific and anti-inflammatory drugs, the use of which was supposed to change the dynamics of the disease. Numerous studies of the comparative use of various drugs with the expected result have shown that, in fact, only hormones, and even then not always, can bring a small positive effect (201-208).

Hormonal treatment often performs an unspoken function of a forced measure and a last resort in critical and unclear situations.

However, the use of hormones in pneumonia in general and in viral, in particular, did not play a decisive role in improving the results of treatment. At the same time, the use of steroids may bring some improvement in critical AP situations (327). The materials of recent observations indicate that during periods of the disease, when the hormonal background of the body is depleted, the introduction of hormones performs a substitutive role, accompanied by a slight positive dynamics. Among other things, it should be noted that the use of corticosteroids in the initial period of COVID-19 pneumonia may worsen the results of treatment, which does not allow them to be considered as a first aid tool (328).

Thus, among the methods of first and emergency care for patients with AP in the therapeutic arsenal of modern medicine, there is not one, the use of which could slow down the development of the disease and make a change in the dynamics of the inflammatory process. Currently, the means of medical care that are intended to provide it in the first place are palliative and supportive in nature, while the main goal and main efforts are focused on countering the pathogens of AP. The flow of patients with viral pneumonia today fills intensive care units by 79% (329,330), but the organization of the treatment process of these patients is still determined in accordance with the etiological concepts of the disease, some modifications of which are presented as new ideas about pathogenesis (331).

At a time when the inflammatory process in the lung is a fait accompli, and the clinic of the disease is caused by a violation of the functions of the affected organ, in modern medicine there is a noticeable tendency to look for a goal for therapeutic efforts at the microscopic level. In such clinical descriptions, you can get acquainted with the virtual representation of those processes that occur (or are assumed) at the level of cells, substances and molecules as a result of the action of certain pharmacological agents. Such works and studies focus on the possibility of influencing individual micromechanisms that are not directly reflected in clinical symptoms, and the effect of the methods used cannot be assessed using direct diagnostic tests.

For example, no matter what detailed study and subsequent description of the effect of antibiotics on the pathogen of AP does not appear as arguments and evidence in favor of the therapeutic significance of these drugs, the very fact of the destruction of bacteria remains beyond the scope of evaluating the results. That is, this fact is taken into account and evaluated, but not directly, but on the basis of integrative indicators, which include not the result of the direct action of the pathogen itself, but a cascade of subsequent disorders that are the body's reaction to this aggression.

So, having prescribed antibiotics to a patient with AP, the doctor does not seek and does not have the opportunity to observe how the drug destroys microorganisms, since this result exists only in a virtual representation or indirect reflection. Therefore, in this situation, standard diagnostic methods act as the main criteria for the effectiveness of the treatment initiated, starting with the assessment of the general condition of the patient and ending with laboratory data and, of course, the dynamics of the X-ray picture.

It is unlikely that in this situation additional explanations are required to understand that even the most effective results of antimicrobial action cannot bring instant results, right? The effect of any medications used should be taken into account not only at the virtual micro-level of their action. It is important to imagine their place in the overall chain of mechanisms in order to understand which links of pathogenesis should react before the reverse dynamics of the process becomes noticeable if the assistance provided is successful. This postulate is especially important in critical situations when the intended calculation for the rapid action of certain drugs remains invisible and cannot be verified by diagnostic tests.

The last remarks make it possible to understand why the selective evaluation of a wide range of drugs in the treatment of patients with viral forms of AP, mentioned above, does not bring the expected results, although the effect of such tested drugs covers all sides of the process: etiotropic, anti-inflammatory, anticoagulant, immunomodulators, hormones. At the same time, the expectation of new opportunities from the practical implementation of more accurate methods of microbiological diagnostics once again confirms the prevailing commitment to the leading role of the pathogen and etiotropic principles of AP treatment (332-334).

If the search for effective care for patients with AP continues from the point of view of etiology, as the main cause in its development and manifestations, then the section of general pathogenesis in the conditions of such an ideology loses its significance. Interpretation of various mechanisms of the process as consequences of pathogen aggression does not require special clarification of the general pathogenesis scheme, since this information can be gleaned from the microbiological characteristics of etiological factors.

The increased role of viruses in the development of acute inflammation of the lung tissue has not changed the strategic directions of finding effective care for these patients. The search for means of protection against the penetration of viruses into cells today is one of the main goals of the expected success. This goal is partially achieved, for example, by vaccination. However, even if the entire set of modern means of such assistance is used to protect cells from the virus, it will give a preventive, not a therapeutic effect. It is quite obvious that such therapy cannot act as a first aid. And what to do when a person is already ill, especially if the situation is rapidly deteriorating?

In order to have a more imaginative idea of why such an approach to the justification of AP therapy is a delusion, it is necessary to try to combine the basic virtual representations of the process with the real clinical situation. For example, what external signs characterize the fact of virus penetration into cells or the beginning of the action of bacteria on the cellular structures of the body? This moment remains unnoticeable and has no special external manifestations, right? Examination of patients and diagnosis of the disease is based on those signs and evidence that appear later. However, such features are already the result of the subsequent integration of a cascade of reactions manifested by common signs of inflammation, such as fever, cough, shortness of breath, etc., not to mention the infiltration of lung tissue.

Currently, one of the important tasks by which success is expected in the treatment of patients with AP is the differential diagnosis of the disease by etiological signs. For example, it is known that the histological picture of bacterial inflammation in the lungs has noticeable differences from viral. But this picture, which can be evaluated and compared on organ preparations using a microscope, in a real clinical situation, when comparing patients with different etiologies of inflammation, has a virtual character and does not show significant differences depending on the pathogen. Therefore, when evaluating the clinical and radiological data underlying these two seemingly different forms of the disease, it turns out that there are no clear differences between them and, despite the difference in etiology, they are manifested by an identical clinic of the same nosology.

To understand the difference in the significance of the etiological factor as one of the causes of the disease and pathogenetic methods of assistance aimed at eliminating the consequences of this root cause, it is necessary to present the most dramatic situation. If a person begins to suffocate from a foreign body that has entered his respiratory tract, then no one will be engaged in figuring out which specific object got inside and blocked his air access. There is neither time nor opportunity for such inquiries. Anyone who happens to be near the victim at the moment will try to help free his airways from the obstacle, without trying to correct the situation by supplying oxygen and increasing the concentration of the latter in the inhaled air, right?

However, if a patient with AP has increasing shortness of breath and lack of air, then such a clinical picture today serves as an excuse to provide him with oxygen, and in case of insufficient effect - to transfer to artificial ventilation of the lungs. Yes, this is absolutely true, and you are absolutely right that edema and infiltration of lung tissue are not a foreign body, and it is impossible to instantly remove these changes even theoretically. But, at the same time, the percentage of lung tissue damage, which is considered as the basis for the development of this type of respiratory failure, may differ significantly in different patients with critical indicators of hypoxemia, right?

Therefore, oxygen therapy is palliative in nature and cannot radically change the patient's condition, since it does not eliminate generalized spasm of the vessels of the small circulatory circle, which actually underlies the violation of blood oxygenation. Instead of influencing the mechanisms of the pathogenesis of the disease, the main efforts are directed against the pathogen, which in this situation does not directly affect the degree of respiratory disorders. And since among the etiotropic agents currently used for COVID-19 pneumonia, there are no drugs that quickly bring the expected effect, and their search continues, then in this impasse, immunomodulators, plasma injections from convalescents and other means of clearly preventive, not curative action are added to testing.

Despite the palliative and auxiliary nature of most options of modern medical care, sometimes with the help of tactical techniques it is possible to achieve some improvements. This, in particular, applies to the supply of oxygen, as mentioned above, when, by changing the position of the patient or using a special cannula, it is possible to increase blood oxygen saturation. However, such selective actions do not affect the main mechanisms of the inflammatory process, do not slow down its dynamics and do not significantly affect the overall results of treatment.

The results of pathogenetic methods of providing assistance in AP, which are focused on the chain of mechanisms and their causal relationship, depend on the time of their application. Inflammation is a dynamic process with a constant complication of its constituent characteristics and the addition of new fragments. Therefore, the earlier the treatment is started, the more expressive the result will be. This circumstance is due to the active development of the inflammatory process and its high sensitivity in the initial period to various kinds of influences. This remark applies to both positive and negative effects. If treatment methods are able to have a stimulating effect on the inflammatory process, then this is most clearly manifested in the early stages of the disease (see Fig. 4-5).

Thus, in order to get a tangible result from the initiated treatment of AP, it is necessary to apply an impact on those factors of the inflammatory process that, by the time of first aid, are the leading causes of the severity of clinical manifestations. During the period of the disease, when signs of respiratory and circulatory disorders prevail in clinical symptoms, etiotropic treatment options cannot bring the expected effect, since the cause of the observed deviations is no longer the pathogen, but a change in the function of the organ under the influence of the focus of inflammation.

Among the treatment methods that appear in the list of proven ways to help patients with AP, both methods that inhibit the development of the process and options that can accelerate its dynamics are presented. In this regard, the choice of first aid methods is the most important decision determining the future perspective. Initial treatment and the timing of its use is literally an opportunity to control the dynamics of the inflammatory process, but in order for the result to be positive, it is necessary to focus in your decisions on the sequence of mechanisms underlying the pathogenesis of the disease.

5.2. First and emergency care for patients with acute pneumonia

First and emergency care for patients with AP is a type of treatment that should be immediately applied immediately after diagnosis. If the first treatment procedures are delayed or postponed, it should be borne in mind that at this time the process continues to progress, complicating the initial conditions, especially in the case of aggressive development. Such delays in emergency medicine have no justification, as they imperceptibly create additional difficulties in the treatment of patients.

The purpose of using such methods is, first of all, the elimination of emerging disorders of pulmonary blood flow and inhibition of the processes of increasing inflammatory edema and infiltration in the lesion. As evidenced by the information presented above about the mechanisms of disorders that occur in parallel with the appearance of a focus of inflammation in the lung tissue, it is shifts in the circulatory system that are the leading cause of the main clinical symptoms and deterioration of patients with AP.

Inflammation of the lung tissue is an autonomous protective process in our body. The potential of such a protective reaction to the damaging effects of various factors is inherent in our body by nature, and the further continuation of such a process follows a single scenario. The onset of an inflammatory reaction occurs automatically, and its features are exclusively individual in nature, which depends on a number of local and general factors. At the same time, the organism lacks the possibility of conscious and purposeful influence on this process, but the intensity of the disease that has begun is determined by a combination of innate and acquired qualities of the organism itself.

A repeated simplified mention of the causes underlying the unique individual manifestations of AP is necessary in this case in order to once again focus on the factors determining the symptoms that are observed in a clinical situation. On the one hand, the body has internal reserves that automatically and autonomously begin their implementation when a danger occurs, but, on the other hand, we do not have the ability to meaningfully control and manage such a reaction. In addition, to date, no criteria have been defined on the basis of which it would be possible to predict in advance and determine the intensity and severity of further development of the disease.

In this aspect, it is quite obvious that the causative agent of the process is not the main and leading factor determining the characteristics of the disease in each case. An infinite range of process variants under the conditions of the same etiology continues to be observed for many years, regardless of the change of leaders among the pathogens of AP. Attempts in such a situation to single out the microbiological factor as the main one and count on success, making efforts to neutralize it, have repeatedly shown the futility of this direction, especially with the aggressive development of inflammation. The failure of such efforts to improve microbiological diagnosis and the use of etiotropic treatment as early as possible was noted above with reference to the published results.

The rapid and aggressive development of the inflammatory process in the lung tissue causes the body to automatically reduce the load on the small circle of blood circulation, saving its own lungs from the danger of increased inflammatory edema. However, in the conditions of the rapid dynamics of the process, such a protective reaction turns out to be "blind" and uncoordinated. The vessels in the lesion of the lung tissue act as a reflexogenic zone, which leads to a generalized spasm of small vessels of the lungs. As a result of obstruction of blood flow in the system of the small circle, there is a violation of the entire blood circulation in the body, which in the most severe situations is accompanied by an increase in central venous pressure, signs of overload of the right parts of the heart, a reflex decrease in systemic arterial pressure, a widespread violation of microcirculation and metabolism.

This mechanism of emerging disorders in the intensive development of AP has already been discussed above. If, in the described situation, venous return increases due to intravenous infusions, this procedure may aggravate the deviations that have arisen. It should be noted that even against the background of intravenous infusions, the body of many patients has additional resources to level such an unexpected load, since some experts recommend careful intravenous infusions to patients with AP, paying attention to the fact that this procedure is often accompanied by signs of overload of the right heart and instability of hemodynamics (39,134,335). It is difficult to determine the criteria for cautious infusions based on such conclusions, given that pneumonia is considered the main cause of septic complications (336-339), in which, on the contrary, it is recommended to force intravenous infusions in the form of boluses.

If we consider such situations from the point of view of the pathogenetic concept of AP, then any intravenous infusions in the initial period of the disease should be excluded from the treatment complex as a method acting against compensatory mechanisms. In case of individual need for intravenous administration of drugs, such a procedure can be performed in the form of an injection into a vein using a syringe with a minimum volume of fluid. The elimination of clinical symptoms, which today are considered as manifestations of sepsis in AP, is possible literally within a few minutes by eliminating the reflex effect of the focus of inflammation on the circulatory system. At the same time, the "fluid deficiency" in the body, which is attributed to unaccounted losses, is restored spontaneously (!) without additional effort.

A description of one of the procedures by which such an impressive effect can be obtained was given above in Section 4.2.4. In this section, not only a description of the CVSB technique is given, but also objective evidence of its successful effect on the functional parameters of ventilation and blood flow is presented (Fig. 12 and 13). We considered this procedure as one of the options for antishock therapy, which was used during the hospitalization of patients with AP with a pulmonogenic shock clinic. CVSB was not the only medical procedure that was tested as a first and emergency aid in the initial period of this disease. One of the widely available and fairly simple antishock procedures is cupping therapy (CPT).

CPT has an ancient history of its origin, which dates back more than three millennia (49). Currently, this method belongs to the category of alternative medicine and receives diametrically opposite assessments - from complete denial of its medicinal properties to laudatory reviews. We can recall the photo of 23-time Olympic champion Michael Phelps with traces of medical cans on his body, which was printed by the world's leading press in 2016. The purpose of this publication was due only to the non-standard nature of such photo information, since the purpose of using cans in a healthy athlete was not advertised and hardly had a serious justification. However, in this context, it is necessary to talk not about the fashion for this procedure, but about the assessment of its therapeutic effect and the expediency of its use in patients with AP.

The wide divergence of opinions on the admissibility of the use of CPT in medical practice and assessments of its therapeutic effect makes us pay attention to the fact that a completely useless and ineffective technique could not maintain its position in the list of medical care for several millennia, right? But, on the other hand, such a range of opinions suggests that no serious and objective CPT study has been conducted. In the available literature there are no clear indications for the use of this technique, as well as convincing evidence of its therapeutic effect.

A method that is considered as a way to treat a wide range of diseases should at least cause caution, especially when it is proposed for a specific application. Today, CPT is perceived by many people, especially medical specialists, as an ancient method of treatment with questionable effectiveness, which does not fit into the arsenal of modern medicine. In the literature, you can find information about the variety of indications for the use of this technique and completely unconvincing materials about its therapeutic effect.

For example, in recent years, CPT has been widely used in outpatient settings as an alternative method of treating various pain syndromes. The evaluation of the results achieved in this case and the interpretation of the effectiveness of this method are very doubtful and unconvincing. Thus, many authors focus only on a subjective assessment of the result based on the feelings of patients (340-343). Other researchers evaluate the result of CPT as a psychological effect or a placebo variant (344,345). The assessment of the dynamics of some laboratory parameters as a result of the use of CPT already looks like an attempt to find objective criteria (346,347).

CPT was a fairly common type of outpatient treatment in the region where our study was conducted. Basically, this technique was used as a treatment option at home, and the main reason for the use of CPT was inflammatory diseases of the respiratory system. This type of treatment has not been used in inpatient settings. Previous experience of using this therapy in patients with AP has created a subjective impression of its noticeable positive effect. In connection with the latter, an objective assessment of the effect of this procedure on the functional parameters of the pulmonary-cardiac apparatus in patients with AP using CRPG was carried out.

CPT was used in the hospitalization of patients with initial forms of AP as a method of first aid. Dry cups were used, which were superimposed on the back area (avoiding the lower back) from an approximate calculation of 1 cup (50 cubic centimeters) per 4 kg of body weight. A burning wick was used to create a vacuum. The maximum number of cans used simultaneously during one procedure for an adult was up to 15-20 pieces. If necessary, the procedure can be repeated after 12-24 hours.

The correct use of medical jars by the end of the session left behind characteristic subcutaneous hemorrhages. The effectiveness of this procedure was evaluated using the same CRPG methodology described in section 4.2.4 above. The initial registration of indicators was carried out immediately before the procedure, and then immediately after its completion. The recording electrodes were located on the side wall of the chest at the level of 3-4 ribs and remained in the same place for repeated registration of indicators. The age of the patients in these studies ranged from 3.5 to 14 years. A total of 14 CRPG studies were conducted after CPT.

The analysis of the results was carried out in accordance with the same criteria and the same statistical methodology that were used to evaluate the data obtained after the CVSB and described above. The most surprising result of the CPT evaluation was the fact that the use of this treatment technique actually completely repeated the data obtained after performing CVSB. The ventilation and blood flow curves recorded after the use of CPT repeated the dynamics shown in Figures 12 and 13. Statistical comparison of the results after CPT and CVSB revealed no significant differences.

The conducted studies allowed us to obtain objective evidence of the positive effect of CPT on the mechanisms of AP flow. These materials not only prevent this procedure from being written off as a history dump, but also give every reason to recommend its further use in this group of patients. At a time when there is a search for effective means of treating AP, and the ongoing therapy does not guarantee the possibility of improving the patient's serious condition, this first aid option can be recommended as already proven, simple, reliable and, most importantly, with a quick positive effect.

The only real surprise is the fact that two procedures, completely incomparable in technique and principle of operation, CPT and CVSB, allow you to get an identical result. This circumstance indicates the need for special studies to clarify the mechanisms of action of CPT. However, now, based on an action similar to vagosympathetic blockade, we can talk about the anti-reflex effect of setting cans in the initial period of AP. In other words, CPT in the initial period of the development of aggressive AP eliminates the shockogenic effect of the focus of inflammation in the lung: eliminates generalized spasm of the pulmonary vessels, returns the circulation of the small circle to normal mode and eliminates the factor stimulating an increase in respiratory excursions.

The effect of using CPT in the initial period of AP development, which was recorded using CVSB, during the clinical assessment of the patient's condition allows us to note a decrease in shortness of breath, an improvement in gas exchange indicators and normalization of systemic blood pressure, if a tendency to hypotension was previously recorded. The noted positive changes after the use of CPT are the results that are currently being tried to achieve with the help of oxygen supply, intravenous infusions and subsequent administration of vasopressors. In such situations, the task is to use CPT precisely in the initial period of the disease, when the development of the process has not yet reached the refractory stages. And here the time factor and the correctness of the procedure become crucial.

Another method of providing first aid to patients with AP was body surface cooling (BSC). This technique was initially used in our clinic in patients with hyperthermia for rapid normalization of temperature and prevention of hyperthermic syndrome. However, in the process of applying this technique for various diseases, attention was drawn to the fact that with AP, unlike other categories of patients, it was possible not only to achieve rapid normalization of temperature, but also to have a pronounced positive effect on the dynamics of the disease.

Additional study of this issue has shown that in the arsenal of folk and alternative medicine, methods of short-term cooling of the body of patients with certain conditions and diseases have been used since ancient times. In the popular scientific literature, one can find references to the fact that in the old days patients with "overheating" and signs of severe respiratory illness were placed in the snow for a while and even dipped into an ice hole. Such procedures were carried out at that time without any control over the patient's condition and his vital parameters.

Currently, you can easily find ads for special devices for whole body cryotherapy (WBC). Alternative medicine clinics around the world offer the WBC method as a restorative and tonic, treatment of various chronic diseases and syndromes, and even for the prevention of viral infections. Such proposals are formed without the results of special studies that could confirm the effectiveness of such techniques. In this regard, the FDA does not recommend the use of WBC for such chronic diseases and conditions as asthma, Alzheimer's disease, fibromyalgia, rheumatoid arthritis, chronic pain syndrome, migraine, etc. (348).

However, WBC is a relatively new modification of reducing body temperature with the help of special equipment. Such equipment and its application have not yet found application in modern medical systems. Therefore, in this case it is necessary to clarify that in relation to the topic under discussion, it is more correct to talk about the technique of general body cooling (GBC), which is used as an emergency in the form of cold wraps or cold baths. This method, borrowed from the experience of ancient medicine, is used in modern medicine very limited. Until now, general hypothermia has been most widely used in clinical settings in neonatology, where it is successfully used for asphyxia and hypoxic threats to the brain (349-351).

Materials on the effect of GBC on pulmonary functions and on pathological processes in the lungs are presented in the available literature rather modestly and among them there is not only clinical, but also experimental information. Nevertheless, the content of such publications should be of undoubted interest to researchers and clinicians in modern conditions. For example, evidence was obtained of the effect of general cooling of the body on reducing the inflammatory response, in particular, in the lung tissue, improving respiratory function and surfactant protection (352-356). In addition to these positive effects, there are reports that in severe patients with ARDS, general body cooling can also reduce the level of inflammatory cytokines (357,358). Unfortunately, the latest reports relate only to individual observations.

In their report on the results of the use of GBC of the body in newborns with asphyxia, V. De Luca et al. (356) note that in patients without signs of lung damage, the anti-inflammatory effect and the effect on surfactant were less pronounced. In this regard, the authors emphasize the importance of further research of this technique and express the hope that in the future it can be used for the treatment of critical respiratory diseases. So far, this is presented in the form of a wish, but our experience of using GBC in patients with AP may already be made public.

Our experience of using GBC in AP at first, as noted above, concerned sick children with hyperthermia. These were usually patients under the age of 5. During the procedure, the patient had to be completely naked, and the cooling itself was carried out with sheets soaked in ice water. The patient's entire body, including the limbs, but leaving the head and face free, was wrapped in such a sheet and smoothed with the palms for better contact with the patient's skin. Cold sheets warmed up quickly, especially at the beginning, and they had to be changed sometimes every 20-40 seconds. The duration of the entire procedure was usually 7-8 minutes, which was determined by measuring body temperature and normalizing it. After that, the skin was dried by wiping, and the patient was placed in a warm atmosphere.

The clinical picture after this procedure has changed for the better to a greater extent than after CPT and CVSB, but, unfortunately, we were unable to record objective evidence of this fact, as was done after the two above-mentioned techniques. In some observations, it was possible to note an almost complete regression of the initial manifestations of AP in the next few hours after hypothermia.

In the future, the use of GBC in patients with AP has undergone changes. First of all, the age of patients has ceased to play a decisive role. In addition, the procedure was initiated for patients without a significant temperature reaction if the initial signs of AP indicated noticeable circulatory and respiratory disorders. Hypothermia was performed on adolescents and adult patients using cold baths with a temperature of about 10-15 degrees Celsius. This procedure also took about 7-8 minutes, but did not exceed 10 minutes. Immersion in cold water should not be instantaneous, so as not to cause negative reflex reactions, which is especially important for the elderly and patients with previous cardiovascular problems.

The GBC technique in patients with AP was used as soon as possible after the diagnosis was confirmed and was performed in patients during the initial period of the disease. The time factor played an important role in such situations, allowing to stop the further development of the process at the diagnosed stage. We considered this technique as a guarantee of future success in the treatment of this category of patients. The procedure was carried out under the supervision of a doctor. Unfortunately, during this work we did not have the necessary equipment to monitor the condition of patients. This section of the work could not be brought to its logical conclusion and confirmed the positive pathogenetic effect with the help of objective tests, but the author hopes that this message will serve as an incentive for further research and practical application of GBC.

As can be seen from the descriptions of first and emergency care for AP, such techniques as CPT and GBC are manipulations, and not drug therapy, which is currently perceived as a more familiar method of treatment. Some exception is CVSB, where an anesthetic is used to block the reflex action of the focus of inflammation. Nevertheless, it should be noted that the timely execution of these manipulations during the hospitalization of patients with AP allowed us to avoid subsequent intubation and assisted ventilation, which, according to the published results, is currently a fairly frequent development of events. The presented methods of emergency care are an alternative to intravenous infusions and oxygen supply, which are usually assigned the function of first aid (359,360).

Infusion therapy in the initial period of AP should be excluded from therapeutic measures as an action that stimulates edema and infiltration of lung tissue in the focus of inflammation. Oxygen insufflation is currently the most common type of first aid, but it is frankly palliative in nature (39,118,157,315-321,361). An increase in the concentration of oxygen in the inhaled air does not eliminate the causes leading to a decrease in blood oxygen saturation. Therefore, even if it is possible to increase the percentage of oxygen saturation in the blood, the general condition of patients is not accompanied by a significant improvement, and shortness of breath and tachycardia actually maintain their rhythm.

5.3. Restoration of bronchial patency and lung reaeration

In the previous sections, materials and evidence of violations of the bronchial lumen during the development of pneumonia were presented. These disorders in bronchogenic inflammatory processes of the lungs are an important link in the chain of morphological changes in lung tissue. The causes of bronchial patency disorders in patients with AP are due to inflammatory edema of the mucous membrane, excess mucus secreted, spasm of the smooth muscles of the bronchioles and their compression by an inflammatory infiltrate. These factors narrow the lumen of the respiratory tract in the area of inflammation up to complete blockade, disrupting drainage and restoration of aeration of the alveolar tissue.

Information about the important role of bronchial patency disorders in the pathogenesis of AR makes it possible to understand the need for methods of its restoration for the overall success of treatment. Without the restoration of bronchial patency in the area of inflammation, it is impossible to even imagine the return of the airiness of the lung tissue and the complete reverse development of the emerging changes. Moreover, prolonged retention of bronchial blockade eventually leads to stabilization of inflammatory changes, which is manifested by obliteration of bronchial communications and the development of fibrosis of the alveolar parts of the organ (201, 202, 204, 205, 262,263,362-366). The direct connection between obliterating bronchiolitis and organizing pneumonia even gives reason to represent them as synonyms of the same phenomenon. However, before permanent irreversible tissue changes occur, this part of the organ remains a vulnerable place, creating conditions for additional infection and new attacks of inflammation.

Among the protective mechanisms that allow the body to maintain the lumen of the bronchi and remove the contents from them, the most effective and effective is cough. This protective reflex also helps to restore the airiness of the lung tissue. As is known about the pathophysiology of this phenomenon, during coughing, the glottis closes briefly with a sharp tension of the respiratory muscles. At this point, the pressure in the airways, which according to Pascal's law spreads evenly in all directions, can reach 100 mmHg. and the speed of the air jet at the moment of opening of the larynx can be equal to 100 miles per hour (247,248,293,367).

Despite such impressive indicators accompanying the moment of coughing, it is necessary to recall that the sensitivity of the cough reflex decreases from the larynx zone in the direction of the bronchi and disappears at the level of small bronchial branches (368). The latter fact explains that in patients with AP in the absence of diffuse bronchitis, cough is not a clear sign. Such a clinical picture, when cough may be absent in patients with AP, form the opinion that endobronchial factors are not of serious importance in the pathogenesis of the disease, and on this basis therapeutic methods of bronchial recanalization are not considered as an important section of medical care.

The same can be noted when coughing with respect to the speed of the air jet, which in the distal parts of the bronchial tree is significantly inferior to this indicator at the level of the larynx, and therefore the effectiveness of coughing efforts at the level of small bronchi is insignificant. In this regard, D.L.Tuna et al. (369) quite reasonably note that in order to enhance the effect of this protective reaction, its repeated repetition is necessary with a simultaneous decrease in the viscosity of the contents of the bronchi.

If we rely on information about the morphology and pathophysiology of AP, then the most important is the recanalization of small branches of the bronchial tree, which, with acute inflammation of the parenchyma surrounding them, are stably blocked. However, pathophysiological data on cough, as the natural and most active mechanism for restoring the lumen of the respiratory tract, indicate its least effectiveness just at the level of the distal bronchi. In this situation, it is important to take into account not the amount of sputum secreted by AP patients during coughing, which may indeed be quite a bit, but the diffuse effect of a short-term increase in pressure in the bronchial tree. This factor contributes to the expansion of the bronchial lumen and the entry of air into the alveoli, preventing them from filling with inflammatory exudate.

During an active cough, there is also movement in the proximal direction of the contents of the small bronchi. It is this segment of the bronchial tree in the area of inflammation that is characterized by an increased process of mucus formation. The use of means that reduce the viscosity of sputum facilitates its evacuation. The restoration of bronchial patency in the affected area affects the inhibition of the inflammatory transformation of the pulmonary parenchyma, the return of airiness to it and the elimination of changes that have already occurred. The intensity and frequency of such medical procedures require frequent round-the-clock repetition.

Not so long ago, in our recent past, a combination of drugs that dilute the bronchial contents and methods of its active removal by the patients themselves were a fairly popular and widespread method of helping patients with AP. But today, with regret, it can be stated that this therapeutic direction has actually ceased to be mentioned and discussed in publications on this topic, and rare generalizing reports on this section of the problem raise more questions about the methods of evaluating the results than about the effectiveness of the means used.

For example, R. Anand et al. (257) conducted an extensive review of the literature on the effectiveness of mucoactive agents for acute respiratory failure in the critically ill, who were mainly on artificial ventilation. The generalization of this review was the conclusion that drugs with mucolytic action do not significantly affect the clinical outcomes in most of these patients.

The use of drugs of this group at the critical stages of the disease is too late help, so the above conclusion, from my point of view, is quite logical. Mucolytics are an auxiliary tool, not a panacea, which can independently restore the lumen of the bronchi. Their appointment is most effective in the early period of the disease, when the patient is able to use the action of mucolytics by actively evacuating bronchial mucus using bronchial "peristalsis" during coughing. Changing the configuration of the bronchi (diameter and length) during coughing can squeeze out the contents of the lumen, which is especially important for the distal parts of the bronchial tree.

It is completely unjustified to passively expect a result from means that dilute sputum. Under the action of mucolytics, sputum, although it becomes less viscous, but the change in quality is not accompanied by its independent removal from the bronchial lumen.

The process of evacuation of the contents requires physical effort, which can be applied by the patient himself or by medical personnel. The most effective recanalization of the bronchial canal at all levels of the respiratory tract can be achieved by stimulating coughing.

When the patient loses the ability to provide an active cough, the difficulties of bronchial recanalization increase. The use of aspiration through an intubation tube to evacuate sputum against the background of a suppressed cough reflex can help to remove mainly the contents from the trachea and large bronchi, however, such a technique cannot provide effective release of the lumen of small bronchial branches, which play a major role in ventilation disorders, especially in the area of inflammation of the lung tissue. In this regard, it is quite obvious that broncholytic therapy should be used as early as possible in order to achieve its maximum effect for the restoration of physiologically important pulmonary parenchyma reaeration.

Another example of a narrow study of a large problem, where the subject of research is a small link at the cellular level from the pathogenetic chain of the disease, is the study of surfactant therapy of severe inflammatory processes in lung tissue, although many of these works are experimental in nature. The desire to improve the results of treatment of severe patients consists in attempts to deliver surfactant to the tissues of the organ in order to restore the airiness and breathability of the damaged part of the pulmonary parenchyma. Such therapy is not accompanied by the elimination of morphological and functional disorders in the lungs, which are the cause of the destruction of its own surfactant, so it is logical that such efforts do not give the expected results.

For example, Piva S. et al. (370) present the results of the administration of a surfactant dissolved in saline solution during bronchoscopy in patients with ARDS, sometimes noting an improvement in some observations. A.V. Bhansali and A. S. Shah

(371) presented a review of the literature on this issue, which includes materials from both clinical and experimental studies. The researchers tried to deliver natural and artificial varieties of surfactant to the lungs using bronchoscopy, inhalation, as well as by constant instillation into the trachea. Minor improvements in the condition of some patients are noted against the background of the lack of overall significant success of this technique, but the brief conclusion of the authors of the review expresses the hope that in the future this type of medical care can play an important role in improving the effectiveness of treatment of severe patients. with inflammatory processes of the lungs.

Optimism and hopes that the local use of surfactant in severe patients with acute bronchopulmonary pathology of an inflammatory nature can bring success in the treatment of this category of patients give way to a completely different perception of this technique, if we analyze some nuances of the observed phenomenon. Firstly, this therapy is of a substitutive nature and is aimed at compensating for the lost factor of stabilizing the volume of the alveoli, and not at eliminating the causes causing its destruction. In this case, preference should be given to therapy that eliminates the causes of damage to the surfactant. As some studies show, if you simply replace the lost surfactant, then even to achieve minor improvements, it will be required in quantities significantly exceeding the natural need for it (371).

Secondly, the vast majority of reports on the use of surfactant are based on observations of patients who have reached critical stages of the disease up to the development of ARDS and their connection to auxiliary ventilation. In fact, we are talking about the treatment of those patients who missed treatment opportunities in the early stages of the process, and the inclusion of surfactant was one of the ways to rectify the situation and a measure of despair in the face of the fiasco of previous efforts.

Finally, it is noted in the presented publications that in order to achieve some effect of surfactant therapy, there was a need for bronchoalveolar lavage, sometimes with the help of a solution of the surfactant itself (370 371). In this regard, continuing the topic of the emerging blockade of bronchioles in AP and methods of its elimination, a logical question arises: on the basis of what arguments was it decided and proved that it is surfactant that is the cause of some improvement? Most of the injected drug does not achieve its goal due to blockage of the respiratory tract, and if it does, it cannot fully realize its purpose as a result of the preservation of inflammatory infiltration of tissues. A more likely explanation for the positive changes after such procedures is the washing of the bronchial tree and the physical removal of the contents from its lumen.

Despite the lack of logical prerequisites for the successful use of surfactant in severe forms of AP, some experts express confidence that this method of treatment can not only have achievements in the future, but also help create a new treatment strategy for this group of patients. At the same time, the authors of such a forecast base their hopes not on the scientific justification of the action of this technique in relation to the pathogenesis of AP, but on analogies with the results of the use of surfactant in another pathological condition that has completely different causes of its development, incompatible with the problem of inflammation of the lung tissue.

Thus, a group of experts compares the results of the successful use of surfactant for distress syndrome in premature infants with the results of similar therapy in patients with ARDS with acute inflammatory processes in the lungs (372). Noting the absence (?!) of a similar effect in the second group in the presence of inflammation, the authors only suggest that this may be due to a more complex mechanism for the development of identical disorders. The doubtfulness of the future success of a simple surfactant application in patients with AP is due not only to the lack of positive results of the first implementation of this technique, but also to the lack of scientific justification. Similar attempts to solve the problem of AP, based on analogies with other diseases, have already been cited above for the diagnosis and treatment of septic complications.

The above material and its conclusions are an example of a fairly common trend today to seek a solution to the problem of AP by focusing attention and effort on a small fragment of the pathogenesis of the disease, without taking into account its place in the general chain of mechanisms and interrelation with other factors. In this regard, it is necessary to pay attention once again to the fact that the same disorders in the body may have different causes of their origin. It is well known that, for example, a change in systemic blood pressure, an increase in cytokine production or a change in heart rate can be the result of different and not always comparable causes, right?

In the latter connection, the comparison of surfactant losses in newborns and in patients with inflammatory processes is incorrect, since the pathogenesis of disorders in these two groups that led to similar disorders is not comparable in its mechanisms. To expect the probability of success in the second group of observations after a simple substitution administration of the drug looks rather naive without eliminating the main causes of this syndrome. And finally, the whole process of upcoming research is presented in reverse order. Instead of revising the strategy for solving the AP problem in order to conduct further targeted research and determine the principles of treatment, it is assumed that the results of therapeutic testing of surfactant instillations can serve as an incentive for a new treatment strategy. From my point of view, it is impossible to understand the meaning of such a methodology of scientific research.

Clinical manifestations of acute inflammatory process are characterized by rather rapid dynamics and are caused by various mechanisms of disorders. Timely application of pathogenetic methods at the beginning of AP development is important for inhibiting the dynamics of the disease, and the initial treatment package should include a combination of methods aimed at the main and leading links of pathogenesis. Therefore, pinning hopes on the success of one of the methods used and connecting another to it only in case of its insufficient effectiveness is the most common mistake and irretrievable loss of precious time.

Not every patient's body is able to quickly and effectively eliminate emerging disorders without additional help. These circumstances are one of the reasons for hospitalization and intensification of treatment, as well as the reason for an increase in the duration of the disease. If the treatment does not eliminate the blockade of the small bronchi and does not restore the airiness of the alveolar parts of the lungs, then the inflammatory changes that have arisen in them can stabilize, acquiring morphological constancy. An example of such an outcome of inflammatory processes of the lungs can be obliterating bronchitis and organizing pneumonia, which, as noted above, have been appearing in the literature for many years as one of the consequences of acute illness.

Restoration of bronchial patency just refers to the methods of important, mandatory and permanent care in patients with AP. In recovering patients, one can observe how the airiness of the lung tissue returns in the area of inflammatory infiltration, and interpret this phenomenon as the success of etiotropic agents. However, in fact, this process occurs due to the purely physical recanalization of the bronchial branches, which is imperceptibly achieved by the body itself. It is worth frankly saying that at present, periodically occurring non-intensive cough with AP does not belong to the signs of protection and reaeration of the lung, and its maintenance and stimulation, as a rule, are not taken into account in the treatment package.

Returning to the topic of surfactant administration to patients with AP, it should be noted those factors, the presence of which will hinder success. Firstly, a violation of bronchial patency blocks access to damaged areas of the organ and therefore, as noted above, the surfactant is used without much success in quantities even significantly exceeding the necessary ones. In addition, if the alveolar tissue retains morphological signs of inflammation, then the surfactant does not have the necessary conditions to perform its function.

Finally, it is necessary to pay attention to one well-known fact. When a patient with AP begins the recovery period, the most important sign of this phenomenon is the return of the airiness of the lung tissue at the site of the former inflammatory infiltration. The latter sign appears on repeated radiographs and serves not only as an indirect confirmation of the recanalization of the bronchi in this area, but also, most importantly, reflects the stable preservation of the airiness of the corresponding areas of the lung. But, in order to keep the alveoli in a straightened state, a surfactant is needed, which, as is known, is not used in modern widespread practice, is it not? The above X-ray dynamics indicates that the elimination of inflammatory tissue transformation quickly restores the production of its own substance.

It should also be added that one of the main reasons leading to the loss of surfactant and the development of ARDS are violations of pulmonary blood flow. In turn, as is known, the state of bronchial patency determines the nature of blood circulation in the corresponding areas of the lung tissue, since the body tries to maintain optimal proportions between ventilation and blood flow. Bronchial blockade in AP strengthens and supports the causes of surfactant destruction and alveolar collapse, therefore, without removing the airway barrier, it is impossible to achieve complete reverse development of inflammatory tissue transformation.

In this regard, even a superficial analysis of the raised topic about the restoration of bronchial patency and airiness of lung tissue once again draws attention to the close relationship and causal dependence of various mechanisms of the same disease. This circumstance once again underlines the paramount need for clear ideas about the pathogenesis of AP to justify upcoming studies, and even more so when choosing medical care options.

Of all the variety of existing methods for restoring bronchial patency, the simplest, safest for the patient and quite effective is intensive percussion chest massage with an active cough of the patient himself. To achieve an effect, this procedure requires that medical personnel understand its features not so much in the light of medical science as from the point of view of physics. Moderate and varied shaking and tapping of the chest with parallel cough reproduction contributes to a more productive evacuation of the contents of the bronchi.

A coughing attack during the short-term closure of the glottis increases intra-bronchial pressure, which spreads in all directions, contributing to the expansion of lung tissue and preventing the processes of exudation. It is possible to facilitate the evacuation of the contents of the bronchi with the help of mucolytics, but, in general, to achieve noticeable results, this technique requires fairly frequent and round-the-clock repetition, which is a time-consuming task for medical personnel.

In patients who, due to their age or general condition, cannot reproduce an active cough, it is necessary to stimulate it by inserting a soft catheter into the oropharynx, which is connected to an aspirator. Irritation of the mucous membrane by the catheter near the entrance to the larynx causes a coughing attack, and the incoming mucus or sputum is immediately sucked out through the same catheter. This procedure should also be repeated around the clock, at least after 1-2 hours. It should also be borne in mind that a more intense cough is also more effective.

It is worth mentioning another of the methods of restoring bronchial patency, which was used in our previous practice. This method is not common among the options of medical care in official medicine, however, information about the use of such therapy in modern healthcare systems can be found. We are talking about steam inhalations, which today are mainly considered on social networks and the Internet as one of the means of treatment at home. Nevertheless, official medicine also has in its arsenal the experience of using this method, which is difficult to assess unambiguously from the materials presented.

For example, professional reports on the results of the use of steam inhalations in acute bronchopulmonary diseases, which include AP and bronchiolitis, contain very cautious and vague conclusions about their positive effect (373 374). The experience of using steam inhalations in emergency departments of a number of hospitals in the Netherlands led experts to the conclusion that it is inappropriate to continue using this technique in official medicine (375). As a result of the search for effective means of providing assistance during the SARS-CoV-2 pandemic, one of the clinics in Florence (Italy) recommends that patients use steam inhalations, but based on this report, the US authorities warn against using untested and unapproved methods of treatment (376).

As for the content of these publications, it is necessary to pay attention to the following essential points. Firstly, the procedures were carried out using very primitive devices, which affects the quality of the equipment itself and even leads to possible burns (375). Secondly, this method of treatment can give a positive result in combination with other pathogenetic means of exposure, therefore it is extremely important to keep in mind what goals are pursued when prescribing this technique. A simple inhalation with steam can hardly give an improvement without a subsequent cough and the release of the bronchial lumen. Finally, the presented methods of evaluating effectiveness are more focused on the final results of treatment in comparable groups, rather than on testing the technique itself.

Nevertheless, this method of treatment deserves mention due to the fact that during the period of our study it was tested and objective evidence of its positive role in the treatment of patients with AP was obtained. Steam inhalations were carried out in accordance with the original method protected by a patent (377, 378). This procedure was used in all patients with AP, with the exception of critical and terminal conditions. Steam inhalations were carried out as follows.

Water vapor from the boiling vessel was fed through a tube under a special closed canopy, under which only the patient's head was placed. The technical design of this inhaler excluded the possibility of direct contact of steam with the patient's skin and the possibility of burns. In parallel, oxygen was supplied under the frame during the procedure. The duration of the procedure was no more than 10 minutes. Steam inhalation contributed to the dilution of bronchial secretions, which facilitated its removal from the bronchi. Such inhalations were carried out several times a day. Each procedure ended with percussion massage of the chest and, if necessary, suction of sputum from the oropharynx in the manner described above.

Testing of the steam plant was carried out only in a group of adult patients with AP, since we were unable to obtain objective criteria in children due to age-related behavioral characteristics and difficulties with registering the necessary indicators. Among adult patients, this assessment was carried out using comparative (before and immediately after the procedure) recordings of electrocardiography, rheopulmonography and studies of the acid-base balance of blood (379,380). The results obtained made it possible to note that steam inhalation has a positive effect on lung ventilation, improves the ratio of ventilation and perfusion, optimizes the indicators of gases and acid-base balance of blood.

The information we have received about the effect of steam inhalations on the condition of patients with AP is not exhaustive, and a more detailed study of this method, which has a long history of use, would be very useful. However, the materials on this issue, which are already presented in the literature (373-375), show that the results of such studies and the conclusions arising from them depend on the goals set, ideas about the functioning of this procedure and the nuances of its implementation.

In addition, steam inhalation is limited to the stage of the disease and can bring a greater effect in the initial period of AP. The severe condition of patients should significantly limit the use of this method of treatment. The final evaluation of this therapeutic method depends on the testing methodology. The conclusions of the above publications on the use of steam inhalations are based on the overall final results. Information about the direct effect of the procedure itself on various parameters of the patient's body is not provided, which casts doubt on the validity of the conclusions drawn.

In this context, it is again necessary to pay attention to the prerequisites for the formation of different points of view when assessing and solving the same problem. The most probable reasons for such discrepancies have been discussed above. The positive results of the evaluation of steam inhalations using objective (!) tests that we managed to obtain earlier are radically different from the materials on this topic presented in the literature. Previous experience and objective evidence of the therapeutic benefits of this inhalation method suggest that it makes sense to keep them in the list of potentially possible therapeutic methods of AP treatment, at least at the pre-hospital stage. In addition, there may be interested researchers who will be able to continue and deepen the study of this technique.

Methods of restoring bronchial patency are the most time-consuming and difficult part of the work of medical personnel. The need for their frequent and round-the-clock repetition serves as an excuse to search for manipulations that reduce the physical load on performers without losing the quality of the procedures themselves. One of the methods of such therapy that met the above requirements was microtracheostomy (MTS) in our previous practice.

MTS is an aggressive method of restoring bronchial patency. The MTS methodology was developed and proposed by Keown in 1960 (381). A poly-chlorvinyl catheter with a diameter of 0.8 mm under local anesthesia is inserted into the trachea through its puncture under the 2nd or 3rd cartilage rings. The inner end of the catheter was installed at the level of tracheal bifurcation, which made it possible to achieve the most effective stimulation of cough, which was achieved by instilling several milliliters of saline solution. In the case of a deeper location of the end of the catheter in the bronchial tree, the cough during the administration of the solution was less active or did not even occur. In this regard, X-ray contrast examination of the catheter was used to determine the localization of its internal part in a number of patients (Section 3.2.2, Fig. 8).

This more aggressive method of restoring bronchial patency was developed and proposed by Keown in 1960 (381). A catheter under local anesthesia is inserted into the trachea through its puncture between the 2nd and 3rd cartilage rings. Polyvinyl chloride catheters with a diameter of 0.8 mm were used for microtracheostomy. The tip of the catheter was installed at the level of tracheal bifurcation, which made it possible to achieve the most effective cough stimulation. This procedure was performed by injecting saline solution. In the case of a deeper location of the end of the catheter in the bronchial tree, the cough during the administration of the solution was less active or did not even occur. In this regard, X-ray contrast examination of the catheter was used to determine the localization of its internal part in a number of patients (Section 3.2.2, Fig. 8).

Tracheobronchial lavage and cough stimulation with MTS can be performed hourly. This technique is very effective for recanalization of the bronchi and restoration of the airiness of the lung tissue and greatly facilitates work with patients, especially when it is extremely difficult to cause an active cough in them. Most often it concerns children of the first years of life. At the same time, the technique of inserting a catheter into the trachea is quite aggressive, belongs to the category of surgical micromanipulations and requires certain skills to perform it. The latter circumstances can probably explain the fact that this method is not widely used.

In the dynamics of AP development, when the condition of patients becomes severe or extremely severe, their activity and potential to use their own mechanisms for restoring bronchial patency sharply decrease. The sensitivity of the cough reflex decreases, which reduces the effectiveness of the therapeutic techniques presented above.

In such situations, the issue of releasing the lumen of the bronchial tree is often resolved in favor of aspiration of the contents using bronchoscopy. This instrumental manipulation in patients with AP often becomes necessary as their condition worsens, and its performance even by qualified specialists (taking into account general anesthesia, controlled ventilation of the lungs and the inevitable micro-injuries of the mucous membrane of the respiratory tract) becomes a serious test for the patient's body. With the onset of the SARS-CoV-2 pandemic, the risk of this procedure for its perpetrators has also increased due to the likelihood of infection.

Unlike the procedures described above, conducting a bronchoscopy for the patient himself is a passive action that replaces those bronchial cleansing mechanisms that he cannot reproduce or they do not provide the necessary effectiveness. In recent years, indications for performing this endoscopic procedure are signs and conditions such as further deterioration of patients' condition, increased hypoxemia, development of atelectasis, difficulty in auxiliary ventilation, suspicion of superinfection (382-385). At the same time, microbiological examination of the contents of the bronchi appears in all these reports as an important goal of diagnosis during endoscopy, and in other works, the determination of the etiology of the disease was considered as the main indication for bronchoscopy (386-389).

When analyzing modern materials in any area of the AP problem, one can notice the dominant influence of a general strategy that focuses on the etiology of the disease. In this context, the topic of endobronchial disorders in the pathogenesis of AP and the attitude to this factor in the treatment of patients is no exception. The period of the disease and the purpose of using bronchoscopy in the general complex of medical care for this group of patients can serve as another example of the deformation of ideas about priorities among the mechanisms of AP.

Thus, at present, discussions of complex therapy of the early stages of AP actually bypass the use of methods for restoring bronchial patency. The decision to perform endoscopic manipulation is usually made in the late stages of pneumonia, when the process is almost completely out of control. The prevailing hopes for a possible correction of the situation with the help of targeted antibacterial therapy define microbiological diagnostics as one of the main goals of bronchoscopy. Concentrating on the pathogens of the process, experts leave endobronchial findings without proper explanation and relevant conclusions, which are often perceived as an unexpected surprise, but are of undoubted interest for understanding the nuances of the current process.

Many specialists pay attention to the fact that during bronchoscopy in patients with AP, a large amount of mucus and bronchial plugs are washed out of the bronchial tree, although clinical signs before the procedure do not always allow us to assume such results (382-385,390). After bronchoalveolar lavage, the authors usually note an improvement in the condition of many patients. In this regard, bronchoscopy data clearly show that endobronchial mechanisms of disorders are present among the main factors of AP pathogenesis and affect the dynamics of the process, but are not always accompanied by sufficiently pronounced symptoms. At the same time, by the time of the endoscopy, the use of techniques that could be quite effective with their timely application turned out to be unclaimed.

In connection with the latter, it is necessary and important to pay attention to the effectiveness of further treatment after performing one of the main tasks of bronchoscopy - microbiological diagnosis of bronchial contents. The above materials show that the positive results of such studies did not exceed half of the cases, which can be considered as a consequence of successful preliminary etiotropic therapy. The correction of antimicrobial treatment carried out on the basis of the obtained analyses did not significantly affect the final results. Moreover, sometimes the bacterial flora in such patients is determined only in a quarter of observations, and the data obtained also do not affect the results of subsequent therapy (387,391).

Thus, the main conclusion that follows from this small section is quite obvious. Violation of bronchial patency in AP is one of the constant signs of inflammatory transformations of lung tissue. The direct dependence of ventilation and pulmonary blood flow on the state of the respiratory tract translates bronchial blockade into the category of important factors supporting the inflammatory process. Without restoring the drainage function of the bronchial tree, it is impossible to eliminate the inflammatory transformation of lung tissue. The stability of bronchial blockade contributes to the processes of organization in the area of inflammation. Methods of active bronchial recanalization are an important and mandatory section of the pathogenetic therapy of AP, and the options and intensity of their use should be determined by the individual characteristics of the course of the disease.

5.4. Auxiliary and additional means of conservative treatment of acute pneumonia

5.4.1. Etiotropic means of treatment

Etiotropic therapy of AP mainly involves the use of antibiotics. The widespread attitude towards this type of therapy reflects its priority in the treatment regimens of this disease, which in manuals, monographs and review articles always begin with a list of recommended antibiotics. Such descriptions occupy most of the treatment sections and are more similar to excerpts from pharmacological reference books. The belief in the irreplaceability and exclusivity of these drugs over a long period of their use has gradually turned into blind conviction, as evidenced by the experience of the current SARS-CoV-2 pandemic. For example, now that it is already well known that the coronavirus cannot be a target for antibiotics, they continue to be used much more widely than permissible situations allow (109-116).

The inclusion of etiotropic agents, primarily antibiotics, in the section of auxiliary and additional methods of AP treatment logically follows from the analysis of the facts that the role of etiology in the occurrence of the disease and its influence on the formation of clinical manifestations is not the leading factor. However, the modern interpretation of the nature of AP and approaches to its treatment is based on the opposite point of view. The psychological perception of this problem today has deep didactic roots, and established traditions in this matter will interfere with the necessary correction of views.

The role of the AP pathogen as one of the triggering factors of the process begins to lose its leading importance with the development of inflammatory tissue transformation that disrupts the function of the affected organ. It is the latter circumstance that determines the specifics of the disease, therefore, the exclusively antimicrobial effect of etiotropic drugs in such a situation can no longer be considered as the main therapeutic aid.

The importance of microflora in the development of AP and its complications, as well as the effectiveness of antimicrobial therapy in this disease can be most accurately and reliably traced on the basis of EP statistics due to the following features. Firstly, this complication of AP is considered to be the result of infection of the pleural cavity and is considered as a consequence of ineffective antimicrobial treatment at previous stages of the disease. Secondly, the occurrence of EP allows for a microbiological study of the material directly from the inflammation zone in all patients of this group, which is important both for obtaining information about the etiology of the process and for evaluating previous antibacterial treatment.

According to statistics, the frequency of EP development has changed markedly in different periods. For example, in the era before antibiotics, EP was observed in 5% of cases of AP, but after the start of the use of antibiotics, this indicator decreased to 2% (270, 392). However, in the 90s of the 20th century, the number of such patients began to grow again and in recent years the frequency of EP is from 5 to 10%, which exceeds the figure that was recorded before the introduction of antibiotics into practice (270, 393, 394).

Examination of the purulent contents of the pleura reveals microflora on average only in half of the observations (271,395-398), which may indicate, first of all, the effectiveness of previous antibacterial therapy, as well as the importance of other causes in the pathogenesis of the development of EP. Such causes that can stimulate the process of exudation in the area of inflammation in AR and create prerequisites for the development of pleural complications were discussed above. In this context, it should be noted that, according to statistics, the results of treatment and mortality rates did not depend on the nature of bacteriological studies of pleural contents (399).

The presented statistical data quite dispassionately show that antibacterial therapy, which continues to be considered as the main therapeutic agent, is not a salvation from the development of EP. Moreover, there is a progression of the disease and the appearance of pus in the pleural cavity, despite successful antibacterial therapy and sterilization of pleural contents. In other words, at least in half of the observations, antibiotics achieve the purpose of their use, but this circumstance does not have a decisive influence on the overall dynamics of the process. This fact is one of the convincing reasons for a serious reassessment of the priorities that prevail today in the complex treatment of AP.

As such statistics of bacterial forms of AP show, the action of antibiotics, even in the case of their maximum effectiveness, is not a guarantee of overall success in the treatment of this group of patients. Can antibiotics be considered the main, and even more so the only means of treating AP, if sterilization of the inflammatory zone with their help does not stop the growing signs of inflammation and the further occurrence of pleural complications?

Not only antibiotics, but also other types of etiotropic drugs cannot claim to be the leading method of AP treatment. For example, the development of viral forms of the disease occurs according to a scenario similar to bacterial pneumonia. This circumstance suggests that even if effective antiviral drugs are developed, they will not be able to neutralize all the main mechanisms of the process and they should be considered only as one of the options for additional and auxiliary treatment.

Another information about the peculiarities of the use of antibiotics gives reason to critically evaluate the widespread opinion about their leading role in the treatment of AP. Thus, for many years, the duration of antibacterial therapy in patients with AP was determined not only by clinical symptoms, but also by radiological signs of the process, and the courses of such treatment were quite long. Long-term courses of antibiotic treatment were justified by information about a decrease in their effectiveness, as well as the emergence and spread of antibiotic-resistant strains.

Against the background of the established tradition of using antibiotics "to the bitter end", WHO recommendations on reducing the course of antibiotics for AP to 3-5 days appeared quite unexpectedly (119). At first, the submitted documents concerned only the treatment of pneumonia in children, but later publications appeared on the results of the clinical application of these recommendations in adults as well (6,116,120, 121,400). This information is very interesting and indicative of its subsequent results, which showed that such a sharp reduction in the use of the "main" means for AP does not worsen the final indicators.

The presented publications should have unwittingly caused a heated discussion on this topic, since the question logically follows from their content: if such a drastic change in the conditions of antibacterial therapy does not affect the quality of results, how much does this type of treatment help in eliminating the inflammatory process in AP? There are no signs of such a discussion reviving yet, but the answer to this question is given in the title of this section, where antibiotic therapy is classified as additional methods of care.

Such an interpretation of etiotropic agents corresponds to their potential capabilities in the general complex of AP treatment. The causative agent remains one of the triggering factors of the inflammatory process and does not have an absolute effect on the manifestations of the disease itself. The development of the inflammatory process generates clinical symptoms that depend on the localization of the focus and dysfunction of the affected organ, but the clinical picture of AP is not a complete reflection of the properties of its pathogen. The etiology of the process cannot be established on the basis of general diagnostic criteria. At the same time, conducting microbiological diagnostics of AP, on which a decisive stake is still being placed and great hopes are pinned, continues to be a difficult practical task, and the results of such studies remain questionable both in terms of their reliability and real benefits.

Such an image of the causative agent of the process has been formed for years under the didactic influence of an overestimated evaluation of antibiotics and continues to determine the strategy for solving the problem, despite the obvious inconsistency and uncertainty of etiology in most patients with AP. The available data indicate that the clinical manifestations of AP depend on the body's response to the inflammatory process that has arisen in the lung tissue. The microbiology of inflammation does not have an absolute influence on the degree of this reaction, which, together with the compensatory mechanisms opposing it, determines the depth of functional disorders of the affected organ.

Investigating and applying pathogenetic approaches to the treatment of this category of patients in our work, it could be noted that the necessary effect of medical care could be obtained fairly quickly and the need to continue the course of antibiotics in most cases disappeared within a week. According to the results of emergency correction at the early stages of the disease of the main pathogenetic mechanisms of AP, positive dynamics was achieved, and the use of antibiotics in such a situation was of the nature of additional assistance. The use of antibacterial therapy in the form of short (5-7 days) auxiliary courses did not prevent the achievement of impressive results (135).

At the time when the above work was carried out, and it was more than three or four decades ago, methods for determining the etiology of AP still did not cause such widespread doubts about the reliability of their results, and the leading role of antibiotics in the treatment of this category of patients was considered as an unconditional and only true principle. Over the past time, the deepening of the consequences of the use of antibiotics has gradually become an occasion for discussion and recognition of facts that have been traced for many years. This has somewhat changed the approach to the use of antibiotics. However, the didactic influence of this type of therapy remains dominant in the strategic direction of attempts to solve the problem of AP at the present time.

For example, experts began to note that the choice of antimicrobial drugs in patients with AP, as a rule, is empirical (2, 6, 7, 15, 59, 60, 325, 387,401-403), which actually confirms the lack of any real progress in the diagnosis of the pathogen compared to the first experience of antibiotic therapy. In addition, recommendations on the empirical choice and combination of drugs that could initially affect all possible and most likely associations of microorganisms began to appear in such publications. Finally, there is a tendency to reduce the courses of treatment with antibiotics.

In this regard, it should be noted that these changes in the modern principles of prescribing antibiotics have appeared literally in recent years, while during our work they were one of the rules for the selection and use of these drugs. The fundamental difference between modern antimicrobial treatment is that it continues to be considered as the main and leading method of first aid. Since antibiotics retain their role and importance among the means of medical care for patients with AP, it makes sense to briefly outline our principles of this therapy.

1. Antibiotics remain an important but complementary drug in the treatment of patients with acute bacterial pneumonia.

2. Antibiotics are exclusively antimicrobial drugs and do not have a direct effect on the mechanisms of the inflammatory process.

3. The selective effect of antibiotics on the microflora does not give grounds to consider them the main, and even more so the only means for the treatment of AP, when the influence of the focus of inflammation on the clinic of the disease exceeds the value of its etiology.

4. Antimicrobial therapy of bacterial forms of AP is a supplement and continuation of the treatment complex after the use of first aid

and emergency care methods, including permanent active restoration of bronchial patency.

5. Modern methods for determining bacterial pathogens of AP in the most important early period of the development of the disease do not provide reliable results of the study, especially when material from other anatomical areas of the patient is used.

6. The empirical choice of antibiotics for AP should be based on the probability of both gram-positive and gram-negative microorganisms participating in inflammation, and not on indirect signs and assumptions about the presence of a certain pathogen.

7. A patient with AP can receive antibiotics intravenously, intramuscularly and enterally, depending on the severity of the condition and the characteristics of the dynamics of the disease.

8. When choosing an intravenous method of antibiotic administration, the volume of the solution should be minimal, and the ideal method is slow injection with a syringe.

9. The optimal duration of antibacterial therapy for AP is a course of treatment for a period of 5-7 days.

In the course of our previous work, the presented principles of antibacterial therapy were used, which in fact do not differ in any way from the currently common approaches to this therapy, except for the role assigned to it. In patients with initial forms of AP, a bacteriological study was not conducted in our clinic, since during this period of the disease it was not possible to obtain material for this test directly from the affected area, and the results of microflora studies from other parts of the patients' body, as noted above, did not affect the choice of drugs.

To date, there have been significant changes in the list of antibiotics used, but during our work, treatment was usually carried out with two or even three antibiotics, the action of which complemented each other and expanded the spectrum of action. Each of the selected drugs was used in the maximum allowable dosages. There was no difference in efficacy between intravenous and intramuscular administration of antibiotics. It should be emphasized that intensive physiotherapy of bronchial drainage continued after the cessation of antibacterial therapy and was always recommended on an outpatient basis after the patient's discharge.

A positive result of the use of antibiotics can be counted on only with bacterial forms of AP, but at present, in the conditions of the current SARS-CoV-2 pandemic, when the number of patients with COVID-19 pneumonia has sharply increased, everyone suddenly felt a shortage of effective antiviral agents. It is this circumstance that is the main reason for the situation of uncertainty and confusion, which primarily engulfed representatives of professional medicine. A manifestation of this atmosphere is the sharply increased number of publications with the results of the search and testing of various antiviral agents, and such materials have begun to occupy a larger volume of many medical journals.

Meanwhile, the reasons for such a passionate search for antiviral drugs did not arise suddenly, as it is perceived in broad sections of society and replicated in the media. For unbiased and objective conclusions on this issue, it is worth recalling at least the epidemiology of AP in recent years before the pandemic. As noted above, at least over the past two decades, many experts have been paying attention to the constant and steady growth of viral inflammation of the lung tissue, which just over a decade ago accounted for almost half of the observations of AP (13). According to statistics provided by S. Jain et al., which CDC refers to in their documents, viral pneumonia in children on the eve of the pandemic accounted for 66% of all cases of AP (404, 405).

Thus, if we focus on information about the dynamics of microbiological factors in the etiology of AP, then the need to find effective antiviral drugs for the treatment of this group of patients has existed for more than one year and, moreover, such a need has not become a sudden consequence of the SARS-CoV-2 pandemic. And if we go back to the results of the two previous coronavirus epidemics (SARS and MERS), it turns out that the current pathogen has been among the virulent causes of AP for a couple of decades.

In recent years, antiviral drugs such as oseltamivir, favipiravir, remdesivir and a number of others have been used without much success in viral forms of AP. The lack of obvious efficacy of such drugs did not cause much concern, since the usual role of the main therapeutic agent was still reserved for antibiotics. In cases where the expected antiviral effect did not manifest itself, hormonal drugs remained a life-saving supplement.

What is happening today with the suddenly increased attempts to provide effective therapy for coronavirus pneumonia is a natural consequence of the dominant etiotropic concepts of AP and repeated trials of already proven antiviral drugs. These searches are permeated with the expectation of drugs active against the coronavirus, and the belief that this step will radically change the situation. At the same time, the results of testing various antiviral drugs show that their use in COVID-19 pneumonia does not give any advantages, and some positive changes were noted only after...dexamethasone (122,198,199).

At the same time, old internalized stereotypes and psychological approaches to the assessment and treatment of AP continue to dominate the COVID-19 pneumonia treatment strategy. No one is puzzled by the widespread but senseless prescribing of antibiotics for coronavirus infection, and in many cases, only suspicions of bacterial co-infection are cited to justify the role of antibiotics in the treatment of patients with COVID-19 pneumonia. Only in some reports one can find experts' concern about this course of events.

For example, B. O'Kelly et al. (110) note that: " *The lack of accurate diagnostics for bacterial infection in COVID-19 and over prescription of antibiotics is likely to have a knock-on effect on the potentially larger and longer lasting global health crisis that is antimicrobial resistance.*" At the same time, the authors, while continuing to use antibiotics and maintaining hope for their former effectiveness, pay attention to only one of the consequences of this type of therapy, which has been an indisputable fact for many years. However, the role of long-term use of antibiotics in changing the proportions and relative activity of various representatives of the microbiological community around us and the undoubted growth of lung inflammatory processes of viral etiology remains virtually untouched. The long-term suppression of bacterial representatives of this community and the constant increase in the proportion of viruses in the etiology of AP is at this stage a postulate about the consequences of antibiotic therapy, which over time and additional study should turn into an axiom.

In this context, it should be noted that there are no real prerequisites to expect the triumph of future antiviral therapy. This type of treatment, in accordance with the nature and mechanisms of AP development, will remain as an additional, not a leading aid. Even if it is possible to obtain an effective drug against coronavirus, its action in the conditions of the patient's body will be extremely difficult. In this case, it is necessary to take into account the fact that the development of the disease begins with the penetration of the virus into the cells. To achieve an antiviral effect, intracellular penetration of a therapeutic drug will be required, which, like a virus, is a foreign substance for cells with unpredictable consequences (475).

5.4.2. Therapy of symptomatic and pathogenetic orientation

In modern conditions, many different medications and techniques are used in the treatment of patients with AP, which are more or less widely used in medical practice, but at the same time they are not specific to this disease, and their effectiveness has no convincing objective evidence or is questionable. Such methods of influence are aimed at correcting certain deviations in the patient's condition or at individual links of the pathogenetic mechanism of the disease.

Among such means of assistance, one of the first that patients with AP receive is the supply of oxygen, which has already been discussed in sufficient detail in previous sections. Here it is only necessary to pay attention to some features of this procedure. Oxygen insufflation is a palliative care method that aims to correct one of the consequences of the disease and does not affect its underlying causes and mechanisms. The principles of operation of this technique are based on a substitutive and supportive action, but do not have a direct therapeutic effect on the mechanisms of the disease.

Oxygen supply to the prone positioning also does not apply to therapeutic methods, but only slightly increases the function of the diaphragm in this position of the body. It is known that the main respiratory muscle in our body is the diaphragm, which provides most of the ventilation of the lungs. In addition, it is also known about the important role of antagonist muscles, which are able to strengthen and maintain the function of opposing muscles. Such an antagonist for the diaphragm are the muscles of the anterior abdominal wall, which in the average patient do not have a good tone and cannot provide high activity of the diaphragm. If you turn the patient on his stomach, the anterior abdominal wall becomes rigid during respiratory excursions, which allows you to strengthen the movements of the diaphragm and increase the volume of ventilation.

If, with the help of various techniques and tricks, it is possible to increase the level of blood oxygenation in a patient with AP, then this is absolutely not equivalent to a noticeable improvement in his condition and inhibition of the dynamics of the inflammatory process in the lung. The development of the disease continues regardless of the oxygen level in the blood, which does not affect subsequent results (319-321).

Compared with oxygen therapy, the use of nitric oxide inhalations in this group of patients looks, at first glance, a more progressive step. It is noted that such inhalations can act as a pulmonary vasodilator, which is already directed against one of the primary pathogenetic mechanisms of the disease. However, the experience of using such inhalation therapy for AP and ARDS did not reveal its therapeutic benefits, while the side effects of this technique with damage to internal organs were quite high (406,407).

It should still be noted that the supply of oxygen to patients with AP and the inhalation of nitric oxide are usually considered as means of providing assistance in the most difficult and far-reaching situations. Therefore, these methods are not among the standard methods of treatment for all patients with this disease. A more familiar and earlier method of helping such patients is the use of various medications with a certain focus of action.

First of all, among the drugs widely used in patients with AP, an extensive group of drugs with anti-inflammatory effects should be distinguished. Nonsteroidal anti-inflammatory drugs are the most available for use in any conditions and are quite popular, but studies in which it would be proved that representatives of this pharmacological group provide significant benefits in the treatment of patients with AP are unknown to us. And although with AP, one of the main signs of the disease is inflammation, and medications such as paracetamol, aspirin, ibuprofen and the like have an anti-inflammatory effect, it is almost impossible to find suggestions for the targeted and continuous use of these drugs among professional recommendations.

The hope for a positive result of the constant use of nonsteroidal anti-inflammatory drugs in AP looks, from my point of view, very problematic, since these drugs can affect only small pathogenetic links in the general mechanism of the disease. At the same time, the side effects of prolonged use of such drugs can create quite serious additional problems (408). In this regard, it is still advisable to use such drugs more as a spare symptomatic remedy, for example, if it is necessary to obtain an antipyretic effect.

Steroid drugs occupy a completely different place in the therapeutic complex of AP and are used more as one of the anti-shock measures than as an anti-inflammatory agent. This group of drugs is usually included in recommendations for helping patients in critical situations or as an option for immunomodulatory therapy in severe cases, but is not a treatment for AP in the early stages of development.

In recent years, and especially after the outbreak of the SARS-CoV-2 pandemic, interest in various immunomodulatory therapy options has increased in the hope of reducing the intensity of the inflammatory response and thereby improving the results of AP treatment. This area of medical care includes the use of corticosteroids, immunoglobulin, tocilizumab, and more recently, plasma from donors who have suffered a coronavirus infection. However, the results of such therapeutic tests do not bring the expected results (149,199,207,208,409-412).

Such tests are usually performed in a group of severe patients, and the observed contingent includes not only cases of AP, but also variants of sepsis and septic shock in other diseases (207,208,409). The choice of the time and stage of the disease is more consistent with the concept of "despair therapy" than the targeted pathogenetic use of such drugs. During the period of the disease, when the inflammatory process has already developed, dictates clinical symptoms and determines the causes of the severity of the patients' condition, relying on immunomodulatory factors is too late a decision. If we proceed from the provisions of the doctrine of the disease, then, for example, the introduction of immunoglobulin is more appropriate before the onset of an inflammatory reaction. This means that such a drug will be more useful for prevention than for the treatment of AP.

In the latter connection, it should be noted that most methods of medical care for patients with AP, including even resuscitation methods such as lung ventilation, which are not only recommended, but also considered as an opportunity for a strategic solution to the problem of the disease, are frankly palliative in nature. It is difficult to imagine how the problem under discussion can be successfully solved by increasing the number of artificial lung ventilation devices produced and increasing their availability per capita. However, it is precisely such actions that are proposed as a strategic solution to the difficulties that have arisen (146-148).

At present, when the complexity of solving the problem of AP has increased due to the increase in the number of viral forms of the disease, the principles of forming common approaches in the treatment of this group of patients are still influenced by the concepts and rules that have been applied and dominated over the past few decades. Only earlier such approaches had a concrete expression when the treatment of AP began according to the formula "antibiotics alone", but if the disease continued to progress, therapy was gradually supplemented with new ways of providing assistance. Now, with COVID-19 pneumonia, antibiotics have lost their usual characteristic of the leading agent, and projects and ideas for finding an equivalent replacement have remained true to the previous concept of the disease.

Attempts to find a new etiotropic panacea do not take into account the pathogenesis of the disease, therefore, the results obtained as a result of testing various drugs are initially focused on the lack of planned success. In the list of modern means and methods of providing care to patients with AP, there are virtually no options for providing care that could have an impact on the process already during its development. The lack of effective first aid and emergency care in the therapeutic arsenal of this group of patients is the reason for the gradual addition of palliative and supportive techniques during the development of the disease, and the principles of such therapeutic approaches do not provide reliable guarantees of success.

5.5. Special assistance in the development of complications in the focus of inflammation

In this section we are talking about complications that are one of the late and severe stages of the development of inflammation in the lung tissue, and their appearance requires the use of additional specific manipulations and methods of medical care.

5.5.1. Principles of treatment of pleural complications

Involvement in the process of the pleural cavity may occur at different times from the onset of the disease. Sometimes, even at the first examination of a patient with AP, signs of thickening of the pleura or even the presence of an effusion in the pleural cavity are revealed. Such radiological symptoms indicate the aggressive nature of the development of the inflammatory process in the lung, reflecting the intense dynamics of the increase in edema and infiltration of tissues in the area of inflammation.

In the old classifications of the disease, such a scenario of the development of inflammation of the lung tissue was attributed to the croup forms of AP. The onset of inflammatory changes in the pleural leaves is usually accompanied by a pain syndrome, which increases with the deepening of respiratory excursions with localization in the side on the side of the lesion or with the irradiation of pain in the abdominal area, which complicates differential diagnosis.

If the patient has the described signs, immediate application of the first and emergency care methods listed above is required. The delay in the provision of these types of medical care is a serious omission, since the inflammatory process continues its pace of development and it is important at what stage it will be applied "inhibitory" therapy. Only after these emergency procedures should additional methods of evacuation of pleural effusion be used, if there is a need to perform this procedure.

In all cases where there are signs of pleural effusion, and its radiological assessment indicates an accumulation of 1 cm or more thick, immediate diagnostic and therapeutic puncture of the pleura is necessary. The performance of this manipulation is desirable in the conditions of local infiltration anesthesia, which greatly simplifies its implementation and is easier to tolerate by the patient. Preliminary execution before the procedure on the side of the CVSB lesion will further facilitate the patient's upcoming manipulation.

The diagnostic value of pleural puncture is due to the fact that only the extraction of pleural contents allows you to study it and accurately determine its nature. The appearance of an effusion in the pleural cavity changes the anatomy of this area and, accordingly, functional parameters, increasing intra-thoracic pressure. Consequently, the therapeutic value of performing a pleural puncture is to release the patient's lung from compression by the surrounding fluid and return the possibility of maximum permissible respiratory excursions. The performance of this therapeutic manipulation should not depend on the intended nature of the contents of the pleura.

If the pleural fluid is serous and is easily evacuated through a puncture needle, then physical extraction of the exudate and further observation will be sufficient. However, if the effusion in the pleural cavity has a fibrinous character and is characterized by a thick consistency, and even more so corresponds to the concept of EP, then the decision on further therapeutic tactics should be taken in favor of drainage. At the same time, the diameter of the tube selected for drainage should be the maximum possible in this situation. The use of thin catheters to provide a more gentle approach discredits the essence of this procedure, since such drains often cease to perform their function in conditions of dense effusion and require replacement with a larger diameter drainage.

Thus, according to various sources, in patients with purulent exudate, drainage blockage is observed with a frequency of 11 to

64%, which forces the replacement of the drainage tube, which has become non-functional, turning simply into a foreign body (270,413,414). In such situations, the possibility of permanent adequate removal of pleural contents is missed, and the delay of thick exudate in the pleural cavity is accompanied by an increase in its concentration due to the gradual absorption of the liquid part and the formation of loculations.

Preferences given to small-diameter pleural drainage up to the insertion of a catheter into the pleural cavity by the Seldinger method are explained not by its functional capabilities, but by less discomfort for patients and are sometimes accompanied by additional administration of fibrinolytics into the pleural cavity. However, proponents of this approach to drainage of the pleural cavity in EP note that this method does not always achieve its goal and in the future there may be a need for surgical means, such as VATS and open thoracotomy with lung decortication (243,270,273, 276,277,415-418).

In recent years, interest in surgical methods of treating EP has increased again, which is due not only to the continued increase in the number of these complications in AP, but also to the problems noted above with the adequacy of drainage of the pleural cavity. Against the background of this trend, no one pays attention to the fact that the desire to reduce discomfort when choosing drainage in a number of patients turns into the need for surgical intervention. Agree that this is far from the best "lottery" to get on the operating table as a result of drainage defects, but the main explanation of this phenomenon, which is currently observed, continues to correlate with the etiology of the process and the shortcomings of etiotropic therapy, sidelining the problem of incomplete evacuation of purulent exudate.

The most rational and justified approach to the application of additional methods of evacuation of pleural effusion are the principles that we have adhered to in our work and which some experts recommend as optimal. Firstly, there is no scientific justification for waiting tactics and abstinence from diagnostic puncture of the pleural cavity, since it is impossible to determine the nature of the effusion without its direct examination (244,270). Secondly, the permissibility of EP treatment with repeated punctures of the pleura does not provide sufficient evacuation of purulent contents and creates prerequisites for the subsequent use of surgical aids (243,273). Finally, if drainage is necessary, a tube of sufficiently wide diameter should be immediately selected, since the properties of purulent exudate do not depend on the anatomical size of the patient (413).

Currently, during the evacuation of pleural exudate, the tendency of gradual transition from more gentle to more aggressive methods is one of the reasons for the preservation of parapneumonic inflammation and the continuing need for surgical interventions. The main source of these complications and the cause of their duration remains the main focus in the lungs, and the success of their elimination depends on the timing of the start and the general principles of treatment. For example, as noted above, intravenous infusions contribute to the preservation of exudation into the pleural cavity, at the same time, etiotropic therapy, despite the existing belief in its crucial importance for eliminating pleural changes, does not bring obvious success, although its action eliminates pathogenic microorganisms in purulent pleural exudate in at least half of the observations.

The occurrence of pyopneumothorax in AP is one of the most urgent situations in the development of this disease. This complication is a consequence of the rejection of necrotic areas of lung tissue into the pleural cavity, where the presence of air indicates the appearance of communication of air-bearing structures with the parapulmonary space. In such situations, discussion of methods of assistance is inappropriate, since when air appears in the pleural cavity, this is often accompanied by the development of a valve mechanism and the danger of intra-thoracic tension syndrome.

It should also be borne in mind that the rejection of necrotic tissues into the pleural cavity can occur in several stages, which is accompanied by a change in the nature of communications between bronchial structures and the pleural cavity. Such a cleansing mechanism in the affected area of the lung can change the conditions that support the pyopneumothorax. For example, some time after the occurrence of pyopneumothorax, the patient may have signs of the formation of a broad bronchopleural fistula or the formation of a valve mechanism. To avoid the suddenness and danger of such situations, when diagnosing air in the pleural cavity in patients with AP, even if there is a doubtful amount of fluid, urgent drainage is necessary.

The development of pneumomediastinum and pneumopericardium is based on other causes of origin, unlike pyopneumothorax. The origin of these complications has been described above, and the microtraumas that cause them explain their more favorable course. Usually these complications do not require urgent application of drainage procedures, which is especially typical for pneumopericardium.

However, when air appears in the mediastinum, constant monitoring of the patient's condition is necessary, since sometimes there is a need for drainage. Such deterioration may be associated with the development of the valve mechanism and further injection of air into the mediastinal tissue with the appearance of signs of increased intra-thoracic pressure. An external sign of such dynamics is an increase in subcutaneous emphysema in the neck, upper chest and face. In this case, an urgent suprajugular mediastinotomy may be required. Signs of increasing cardiac tamponade in the pneumopericardium can be eliminated by puncturing the pericardium at the point between the xiphoid process of the sternum and the left costal arch and, if necessary, drainage by the Seldinger method.

5.5.2. Radical operations in patients with acute pneumonia

The name of this section among the materials about the disease, which is not a constant subject of attention of surgeons, may look quite unexpected and strange. Discussion of the topic of radical operations at a time when methods of gentle surgery in the treatment of complications of AP, such as VATS, have become widespread, seems inappropriate and difficult to explain. However, in this context, we are talking about that rather rare and extremely severe category of patients with AP, for whom the only chance of salvation is timely radical surgical intervention.

Usually such complications and methods of their treatment are discussed in separate publications in surgical journals, and it is not accepted to include such material in the general description of the disease because of its rarity and non-standard. At the same time, mentions of such consequences of AP are most often explained by etiological features. However, in accordance with the doctrine of the disease and the peculiarity of the pathogenetic mechanisms of the development of the process, such forms of lesion should be presented as one of the possible variants of its development, reflecting its most aggressive and severe variety.

In this section we are talking only about one of the forms of damage in AP, which is more often called lung gangrene (LG). There is no complete consensus in the literature on this issue, since various variants of necrotic changes in the lungs are considered under this term. Defining the meaning of the term "lung gangrene", in our work we approached this interpretation from clinical and anatomical positions, which ultimately facilitated the choice of practical solutions. Consequently, LG refers to a complete necrotic lesion of at least one of the lobes of the lung or less often the whole organ.

Such a volume of damage that cannot be repaired makes attempts to correct the situation with the help of conservative treatment meaningless, and the inevitable course of subsequent events at the stage of rejection of necrotic masses puts the issue of early surgical intervention on the agenda. The experience accumulated to date in various clinics shows that it is with LG that conservative methods of treatment invariably fail, while radical surgery is able to save the lives of such patients. In this regard, a wide range of specialists involved in providing medical care to patients with AP should be oriented in the issues of diagnosis and therapeutic tactics for LG.

In the terminology of irreversible lung tissue lesions in AP, the so-called necrotic pneumonia often appears under the diagnosis of "lung gangrene". There are no fundamental differences in the form of the lesion in this case, since in these variants we are talking about necrosis of organ tissues. The difference lies only in the volume of the lesion, on which the subsequent process of liberation of this zone from necrotic masses and the new anatomical variants that arise at the same time depend.

For example, R. Harrington (419), considering various options for the destruction of lung tissue in AP, among which LG appears, gives a description of their pathogenesis with pulmonary and bronchial vascular thrombosis. Possible, according to the author, necrotic complications are presented depending on the possible pathogens of the disease, but there is no complete lesion of the entire organ share in this list.

In other reports, where the analysis of severe necrotic lesions of the lung tissue in AP is given and the term LG appears, according to the presented descriptions of observations and visual illustrations, not in all cases it may be a total lesion of the lung lobe (282-284,420,421).

Multiple, but separate zones of necrosis in the lung, occupying a sufficiently large volume of the organ, are also a very severe form of lesion, but in their consequences they differ significantly from LG. The use of radical lung resections in patients with multiple necrosis zones, as well as in the case of LG, allows 80% of patients to successfully overcome the critical period of the disease (283).

Unfortunately, radical operations do not always bring a positive result, since the timing of such interventions is too late, the patient's body is extremely weakened by this time, despite prolonged intensive therapy, and the pleural cavity, as a rule, is in conditions of persistent purulent inflammation (420,421).

In order to reduce the intensity of inflammation in the pleural cavity and improve conditions for subsequent lung resection, Y. Refaeli and D. Weissberg (422) successfully operated on two patients with LG in two stages. Initially, they performed fenestration of the pleural cavity, and a week later, when the space around the lung was cleared, they were able to perform anatomical resection of the lung.

In order to determine the degree of necrotic changes in the lung and at an earlier date to decide on the feasibility of radical intervention, B. A. Reimel et al. (423) used computed tomography with contrasting pulmonary vessels. Having found preserved diffuse blood flow in the lung tissue with the presence of necrotic cavities, they found no indications for surgical intervention and continued conservative therapy with positive results.

In general, it can be noted that LG is a formidable variant of the development of AP and requires early recognition and urgent surgical intervention. However, the rarity of this form of the disease makes it unfamiliar to a wide range of doctors and makes it difficult to collect information about the clinical and radiological features of LG. In this regard, it is advisable to present our small experience of working with such patients.

In this case, we are talking about a small (11 people) group of children aged the first five years, who accounted for only 1.1% of the total number of patients with AP treated in our clinic. The onset of the disease in these patients resembled other cases of aggressive AP development. However, one of the first signs of irreversible and extensive damage to the lung tissue was the nature of the patient's reaction to first aid and emergency procedures. If in most cases, after the use of these methods, there was a noticeable improvement in the condition of patients, then in those situations when the diagnosis of LH was subsequently confirmed, the result was unstable and short-term.

On the first picture of the chest, sometimes literally in the first hours of the disease, it was possible to detect a massive uniform shading of one of the lobes of the lung. At the same time, the affected lobe had noticeably convex contours and enlarged dimensions, which was a reflection of its pronounced edema and infiltration. An effusion quickly appears in the pleural cavity, which was identified as hemorrhagic during pleural puncture. This type of effusion is usually inherent in a lung infarction. Primary bacteriological examination of pleural fluid, as a rule, did not reveal microflora.

During our work, we did not have the opportunity to investigate any biomarkers or other additional diagnostic methods to clarify the nature of changes in the area of inflammation. Therefore, the main importance was attached to clinical and radiological data. The stable and severe general condition of the patient and the absence of any positive radiological dynamics, despite the intensive use of pathogenetic methods of medical care, served as the basis for standard chest tomography, since at that time we did not yet have computed tomography. Layered images of the chest organs revealed a uniform enlargement and compaction of one of the lobes of the lung with the presence of small irregularly shaped cavities that were not noted on conventional radiographs.

Persistent preservation of the general intense darkening of the entire lobe of the lung with the appearance of small cavities against this background after several days of intensive drainage of the bronchi served as an indirect sign of necrotic changes. The ineffectiveness of conservative treatment in combination with X-ray data and the nature of pleural effusion was regarded as total necrosis of the lung lobe. This conclusion served as a reason for radical intervention. It should be noted that delay in such situations with the provision of surgical care may deprive the patient of the only chance for a favorable outcome.

One of our observations is given as an example of successful treatment of lung gangrene.

The boy is 2 years and 4 months old without any problems in the medical history. Signs of a mild respiratory illness (runny nose and a slight cough without sputum and fever) have been observed in him over the past few days. A sharp deterioration in the child's condition occurred 12 hours before admission to the clinic: the temperature rose to 40 degrees, there was moaning breathing and pain in the left side. AP with a total lesion of the lower lobe of the left lung was diagnosed at the time of admission to the clinic. Started treatment (CVSB, microtracheostomy and continuous stimulation of cough, antibiotic therapy with broad-spectrum actions) have had only short-term effect. The child's condition remained serious. A hemorrhagic effusion appeared in the left pleural cavity. The lower left lobe remained heavily shaded and enlarged on x-rays. The left thoracotomy was performed on the 3rd day after emergency hospitalization. Total necrosis of the left lower lobe was detected (Fig. 14) and its resection was performed. Favorable postoperative period. Recovery.

Additionally, it should be noted that the hemorrhagic effusion obtained during the puncture of the pleura before the operation was sent for bacteriological examination. The result obtained only on the third day of the postoperative period was negative. Histological examination of the removed lobe revealed a picture of total necrosis of all its structures, with the exception of the initial sections of the lobar bronchus. Targeted microscopic examination of the tissue also did not reveal the presence of microorganisms in it.

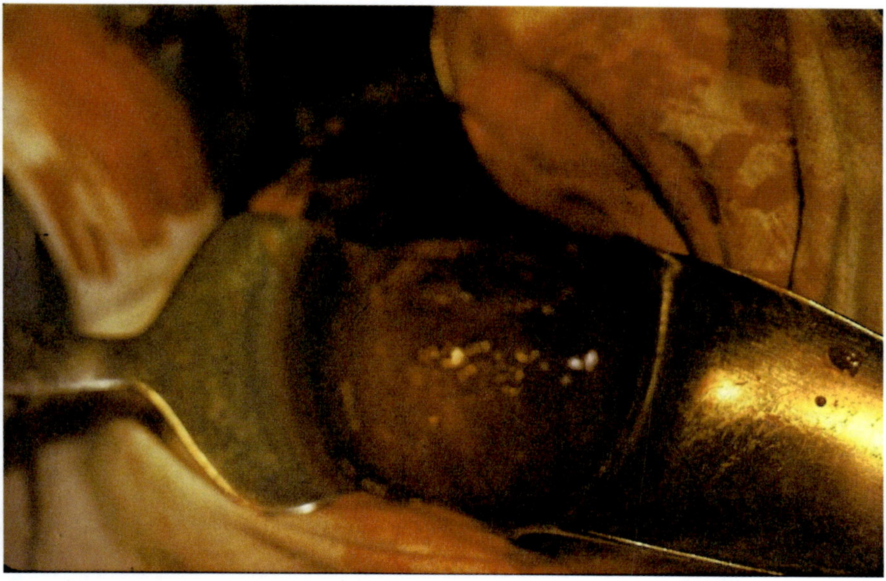

Figure 14. Thoracotomy with gangrene of the lung. The necrotic (black) lobe of the lung is visible in the wound.

Successful surgical treatment was performed on 7 patients hospitalized in our clinic at the beginning of the disease. An analysis of the features of these observations allows us to note that the disease proceeded according to the type of acute infarction of the entire lobe with the lightning-fast development of irreversible tissue changes. Relatively rapid diagnosis of LG and timely successful implementation of the surgical manual allowed to avoid subsequent purulent complications, long-term conservative therapy and quickly stabilize the condition of these patients. In all these cases, the postoperative period proceeded smoothly with a quick recovery and discharge home.

All attempts at conservative treatment of this form of lesion among our observations were unsuccessful. There were also only lobar processes among them, and there were no cases of segmental necrosis or damage to the entire lung. 3 patients with LG were brought to our clinic from other hospitals in terminal condition after unsuccessful conservative treatment. Another observation of this pathology was in the initial period of our work, when the delay in the diagnosis of gangrene and surgical intervention did not allow us to correct the situation in the future. All these 4 cases ended in death.

Currently, the facts about severe necrotic lesions of the lung tissue in coronavirus infection are already known. If at the beginning of the SARS-CoV-2 pandemic opinions were expressed about a "new disease with clinical uncertainty" (42), then as the timing of this catastrophe increases and experience and facts accumulate, it becomes increasingly obvious that we are talking about another outbreak of viral pneumonia, only now on a much larger scale than previously observed. The symptoms of this type of lung inflammation and the nature of the observed complications are difficult to distinguish from similar manifestations of bacterial forms of the disease, which is directly or indirectly confirmed by many researchers and experts.

The similarity of the manifestations of bacterial and viral inflammation in the lungs has been discussed in sufficient detail in the previous sections. Here it is only necessary to consider some nuances of pulmonary and pleural complications arising from COVID-19 pneumonia.

Now that the details of the manifestations of COVID-19 pneumonia have been published, it can be noted that the defeat of lung tissue by coronavirus has many common signs with bacterial forms in the development of complications of the process. For example, many clinicians pay attention to the fact that the appearance of pleural effusion is usually observed in patients with severe disease and is a poor prognostic sign (424). Such a conclusion, according to the AP doctrine, is completely natural, since the appearance of effusion in the pleural cavity is inherent in the most aggressive forms of inflammation. However, the concept of the leading role of the pathogen continues to shift ideas about the causes of pleural complications and the severity of the main process towards its etiology (425).

The intensity of inflammation of the lung tissue in various viral etiologies, including COVID-19, is characterized in the most rapid cases of development by the appearance in the pleural cavity of such an unfavorable type of effusion as hemorrhagic. The frequency of parapneumonic pleurisy reaches 62.5% in viral pneumonia, but how many of them are with hemorrhagic exudate is not specified, since the analysis of such observations is often focused on the results of clinical and radiological examination methods (424). Probably, the frequency of hemorrhagic pleurisy in patients with SARS-CoV-2 is quite high, since the cause of such a pleural reaction is considered to be frequent thrombosis of small pulmonary vessels in combination with hemorrhages in the lung tissue (425-428).

The use of angiocomputer tomography in patients with COVID-19 pneumonia reveals pulmonary vascular thrombosis in 50% of cases (429), and in postmortem studies, thrombosis of small pulmonary vessels is usually the most common finding (429,430). It should be emphasized that mainly the study of the nature of lung tissue damage in SARS-CoV-2 occurs during autopsies, and lifetime diagnosis of necrotic changes in the lung more often occurs in the later stages of the disease.

If we take into account the nature of the pathological transformation of pulmonary structures in coronavirus lesions and the frequency of such findings, we should expect a significant increase in severe necrotic forms of inflammation, which may potentially require surgical care. However, real statistical materials show that necrotic forms of COVID-19 pneumonia are observed with the same frequency as with bacterial CAP variants, not exceeding 4-4,5% (429,431-433).

And yet, extensive necrotic lesions of the lung tissue in coronavirus pneumonia and even lung gangrene are already real complications of this variant of AP, and surgical interventions have not spared this contingent of patients. Surgical interventions for COVID-19 pneumonia are presented as a forced variant of invasive care and are performed in the late period of the disease, when the rejection of necrotic areas of the lungs begins and intensive therapy in combination with the introduction of drains does not bring success.

The description of individual cases of lobectomy and lung decortication in patients with SARS-CoV-2 shows that the indication for surgical intervention was extensive necrotic changes in the lung with pleural complications, including bronchopleural fistula (434,435). The greatest surgical activity in the treatment of patients with COVID-19 pneumonia was demonstrated by A. Hidron et al. (429), who presented an analysis of 19 own observations conducted using various surgical methods. However, the authors included in this group not only lobectomies and lung decortication, which accounted for half of the material, but also drainage, and the total postoperative mortality was 75%.

All these materials, starting with the features of pleural effusion in viral pneumonia and ending with the performance of surgical interventions, were presented in order to show how indications for operations are formed and at what stage of the disease they are currently being carried out. In fact, the published materials from modern clinical experience are devoted to the so-called operation despair, which during the entire period of the surgical specialty were not only the last chance for patients, but also the result of missed opportunities at previous stages of the disease.

On the one hand, many experts note that necrotic forms of lung tissue damage in coronavirus infection are the result of intense and rapid inflammation and hemorrhages (425-428,436), which is most likely at the very beginning of the disease, when blood flow to the inflammatory zone increases and the mechanisms of edema and infiltration actively develop. On the other hand, such a characteristic sign of a severe inflammatory process in the lung tissue as pleural effusion is usually registered 5-7 days after the patient's hospitalization and is considered a sign of an advanced disease (424,437-439). In the latter connection, it is necessary to pay special attention to the fact that the statistics of these reports are based on the timing of hospitalization, and not on the duration of the disease, which are completely unequal concepts when it comes to the pathophysiology of the process.

The appearance of pleural effusion after a week of inpatient treatment and the interpretation of such a clinical picture as a sign of a neglected disease automatically raises the question of the nature of the treatment that patients received during these 5-7 days. It is quite obvious that in such situations, the absence of effective etiotropic treatment methods, which are not present in viral pneumonia, is implied. Other medical care options that such patients currently receive are auxiliary and supportive, but the likelihood of a possible negative impact of such methods on the dynamics of the process is not discussed.

It is difficult to imagine that in the conditions of modern standards of medical care, severe patients during hospitalization were left without intravenous infusion therapy, the negative role of which in AP was shown in the previous sections. This method of medical care continues to be widely used in patients with COVID-19 pneumonia, but the negative dynamics of the process as a result of its influence is explained by other factors. Confirmations of the negative role of intravenous infusions in AP have already been presented and discussed in sufficient detail above, but at the moment it is necessary to pay attention to the search for tests for the earliest possible diagnosis of necrotic changes in lung tissue.

Currently, the appearance of an effusion in the pleural cavity is considered a poor prognostic sign of the inflammatory process, but, apart from such a prognosis, no one is trying to find characteristics to assess the damage to the lung tissue that has occurred by this time. The turning point in the interpretation of pathological changes and the need to solve tactical questions about additional methods of assistance arise, as a rule, in the late period of the disease, when the hidden becomes apparent.

When, during the next X-ray examination of the lungs, destruction cavities suddenly (?!) appear in the organ tissue, these findings, as a rule, are of the nature of an unpleasant surprise and serve as an equally unexpected reason to search for an answer to the question: "What to do?". But the reason for this phenomenon did not suddenly appear during the X-ray, right? Irreversible pathological transformation of the lung tissue occurred much earlier, and now the period of the disease has come, when the inflammatory process no longer has undoubted signs of its further spread and the time has come for cleansing and restoration of this zone.

Yes, the appearance of necrotic cavities in the lung tissue requires a rational assessment and an optimal decision on the need for additional invasive treatment methods. Now the possible treatment options will depend on which scenario further events will develop. If the drainage of such cavities in the lung is insufficient, an abscess will form, and if a valve mechanism occurs in the adducting bronchi, then there is a danger of increasing these cavities in size with an increase in intra-thoracic pressure or their breakthrough into the pleural cavity with the development of pyopneumothorax.

In most cases, such necrotic formations in the lung do not require additional methods of assistance and gradually disappear as a result of scarring. However, there is no reason to consider such a result a success of treatment, since we are talking about different variants of the body's reaction and different limits of the development of the inflammatory process. Standard modern treatment of patients with AP at best does not prevent the expansion of the inflammatory process, and sometimes even able to stimulate it. Therefore, it should be assessed as a positive phenomenon that in most cases necrotic changes were limited to small areas of organ tissues.

In this section we are talking only about those rare cases of the disease that were observed earlier and continue to appear at the present time and in which necrotic changes capture at least the entire lobe of the lung. In such situations, the process of rejection of non-viable tissues can no longer go relatively favorably due to the anatomical spread of the necrosis zone. Therefore, if this variant of lung damage was not recognized in the early stages of the disease, then further developments do not bode well. At best, such a prospect implies the likelihood of performing a "operation despair" with a dubious outcome, and in the worst case, only a pathologist will make an accurate diagnosis (241).

If we evaluate the prospect of AP treatment in the light of pathomorphological transformations in the focus of inflammation, then everything ultimately depends on the nature and timing of emergency care, as well as on the accuracy of early diagnosis of the transformation that occurred at the time of initiation of treatment. To date, medical science has accumulated enough information, facts and objective evidence that make it absolutely clear that early recognition of the morphological consequences of the process and the timely use of adequate therapeutic agents and methods can eliminate the disease in the shortest possible time and avoid the development of complications. Such a formidable form of lesion as LH is not an exception in this list, but it, unlike other variants of necrotic pneumonia, requires early radical surgical intervention.

Suspicion of the development of LG should arise in patients with overaggressive and rapid development of AP. The earliest diagnostic signs characteristic of LG are the rapid appearance of an X-ray picture of a complete homogeneous shading of one of the lobes of the lung, often with signs of an increase in the volume of this lobe and an equally early addition of pleurisy with hemorrhagic effusion. An indirect additional sign of extensive necrotic lesion of the lung tissue may be an unstable and short-term effect from the use of the first and emergency care methods described above.

If the patient has several of the above signs, then it is urgently necessary to clarify the state of blood supply to the inflamed lobe of the lung. Such a test requires angio-computed tomography. Complete loss of the vascular network in the projection of the affected lobe does not allow postponing radical surgery. And although we are talking about the most severe form of lung damage in AP, timely surgical intervention in this situation has a significantly higher success rating than in the case of its use at a later stage of the disease.

CONCLUSION

THE MAIN OBSTACLES FOR FUTURE DECISIONS

The above materials on the state of the AP problem were presented in the form of a comparison of different points of view on the nature of the disease, differences in the reliability and objectivity of existing tests and methods of care, as well as in the mode of constant discussion. The fact that these materials contain objective and indisputable, from my point of view, arguments about the existing distortions in the presentation of the main provisions of the problem does not at all mean their rapid revision and correction.

The experience of debates suggests that not every opponent will strive to understand a point of view that does not coincide with his usual views, especially if these views are shared by the surrounding majority. A broad consensus on certain issues, which, despite the existing contradictions, are considered resolved, according to psychologists, is one of the leading factors that turn collective misconceptions into the most persistent and durable. R. J. Baron and Y. D. Eines (478) explain the psychological foundations of common misconceptions using crowdsourcing, and the transmission of such information through the media and social networks is defined by the authors as adherence to "facts" approved by the crowd, or as a phenomenon of " the wisdom of crowds ".

But it is not only the opinion of the dominant majority that makes it difficult to critically analyze distortions and contradictions in scientific worldviews. Even when the shortcomings of the generally accepted interpretations of the problem begin to become obvious and understandable, there remains another obstacle that cannot be ignored or simply bypassed. In this case, we are talking about job responsibilities and compliance with the established requirements in the relevant fields of activity at all stages of training and work of medical personnel.

In the modern world, there are state programs for training medical personnel. In such systems, each medical problem is presented in the light of the existing concept, which is basic and generally recognized. The theoretical foundations of existing ideas about a specific pathology are reflected in the list of mandatory methods of medical care. Such a multi-stage system of training of medical personnel and their subsequent practice is based on regulatory documents that oblige to provide the necessary standard of medical care, but do not allow the use of unforeseen measures.

The existence of certain standards for the provision of medical care to the population is important, especially in developed countries, where compliance with these rules can be controlled by various structures endowed with a certain influence on specific performers. Such instances include licensing authorities, insurance companies, various consumer protection organizations and even law firms. In such a multidirectional control system, the main focus is on compliance and proper implementation of established standards, while the assessment of new information about the disease and the correction of professional perceptions go beyond these limits, which not only do not allow additional practical initiative, but also restrain the enthusiasm of research.

These considerations are given in order to explain once again the main purpose of the presentation of the presented materials. Despite the objectivity and evidence of many arguments explaining the essence of modern misconceptions about the problem of AP, the information provided cannot be perceived and considered as a guide to practical application. The author's conviction in the validity and correctness of the stated point of view, based on research materials on this problem and confirmed by the results of clinical trials, does not imply a quick, much less automatic correction of existing disorientations.

Widespread and unshakable confidence in the perfection of the modern teaching of the AP prevents a critical assessment of its inconsistencies and contradictions. This psychological problem begins to form during the training period and is further fixed by the established requirements during the practice period. It will take time, effort and patience to change the system of views on the nature of the disease, which has been formed over the years, and begin to perceive a number of fundamental foundations of the current process, which are now not given importance. The organizational and legal features of modern society do not allow avoiding broad discussions, various checks and multilevel decision-making. Such a process requires not only time, but also readiness for these intentions.

Taking into account the stated prerequisites, the publication of the proposed materials was intended as information for reflection. Such information is necessary today for specialists working on solving the problem of AP. Highlighting the problem from a different angle will help to understand the reasons for the gradual and prolonged negative dynamics of results and the lack of strategic success over many years.

The author of these lines has no doubt that when a person is convinced by his own experience of the possibility of avoiding unpleasant developments and knows how this can be foreseen in the future, he will consider it his duty and obligation to share these conclusions with others. This is quite a normal and logical thing to do in such a situation, isn't it? Further results and successes will depend on whether others have used such information and, if so, how correctly and meaningfully.

The intention to present to a wide audience the possibility of effective treatment of patients with AP is based on the results of successful clinical testing of therapeutic approaches that were determined during the revision and adaptation to the biological laws of the doctrine of the disease. The subsequent desire to test the possibilities of pathogenetic approaches to treatment and repeat the results should not come from the automatic and "blind" performance of medical procedures. The chosen treatment procedure, which in the initial period of pneumonia can bring a tangible effect, will lose its effectiveness and meaning as the process develops. Therefore, practical implementation should be preceded by mastering the theoretical foundations of the treatment complex and understanding the dynamics of the painful process.

It is quite obvious that the solution to the problem of AP goes far beyond simple recommendations for the practical application of pathogenetically based treatment principles. Ultimately, the choice of solutions and methods of their implementation will depend primarily on the ideology of the disease, which will determine the list of procedures and therapeutic principles. Proposals for the introduction and expansion of so-called evidence-based medicine to improve such a choice (440-442) will not change the idea of AP and, therefore, will not adjust the principles of existing therapeutic approaches and their results.

When, more than 40 years ago, the mortality rate among hospitalized patients with AP in our clinic exceeded 10%, it was perceived as a terrible catastrophe, because at that time no one reported such depressing figures. Today, such mortality rates among patients with AP in hospital settings have already become familiar, since even more unfavorable results are currently an order of magnitude higher (2,28,167,443). The results that were achieved as a result of our work allowed us to talk about the guaranteed possibility of a rapid cure of AP with the early complex use of pathogenetic care, as well as the prevention of complications of the process.

There were no complications or deaths among the representative group of patients admitted to our clinic during the initial period of aggressive forms of AP. Today, the summary statistics of the results of this work will, in my opinion, be less impressive (135) than the possibility of a visual assessment of the dynamics of the disease in the conditions of pathogenetic treatment. An example of individual observations allows us to give the features of the onset of AP and the X-ray picture at the time of hospitalization. At the same time, each specialist can draw parallels with observations from his own experience and compare the results. To illustrate the above, we offer one of the typical examples from the previous work.

A healthy 22-month-old girl has been showing signs of mild respiratory illness for the past few days without changes in well-being and temperature reaction. Against this background, the day before going to the clinic, there was a sharp deterioration in the condition with hyperthermia, increased cough and shortness of breath. Shortly before hospitalization, she began complaining of abdominal pain. Preliminary treatment was not carried out.

At the time of hospitalization, massive bilateral pneumonia with a slight thickening of the pleura on the left was diagnosed (Fig. 15). Immediately, the patient underwent a vagosympathetic blockade on the left, which was repeated 2 hours later on the right side. For subsequent washing of the tracheobronchial tree and stimulation of cough, microtracheostomy was performed and steam inhalations were additionally prescribed. Cough stimulation was performed with a frequency of once every 2 hours. No bacteriological study was conducted. Antibacterial therapy included intramuscular injections of penicillin and streptomycin in age-related dosages.

After the start of treatment, the patient's condition improved significantly, the pain syndrome disappeared, the body temperature normalized. After 5 days of treatment, there was a complete resolution of the process in both lungs (Fig. 16). After the results of the control X-ray, no further antibiotic treatment was carried out. The girl was discharged home with a recommendation to continue the procedures for draining the bronchial tree.

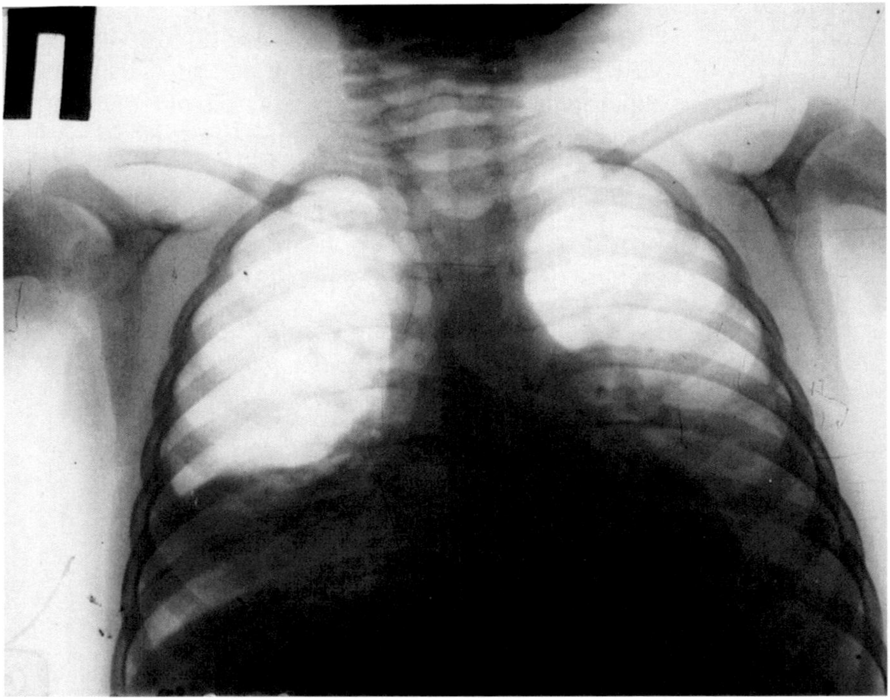

Figure 15. X-ray of a 22-month-old patient, 24 hours after the first signs of AP appear. Intense uniform shading in the basal sections of both lungs with moderate thickening of the pleura on the left.

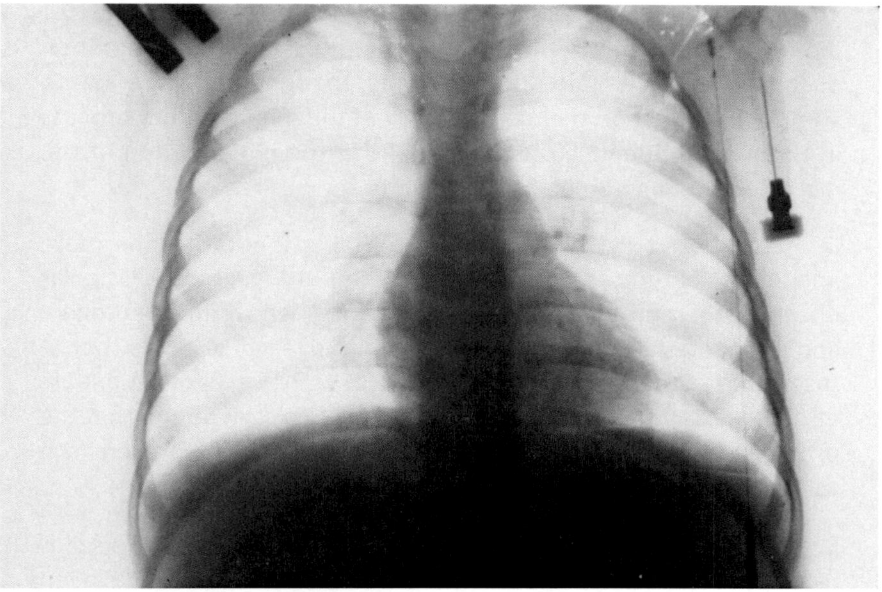

Figure 16. X-ray of the same patient (see Figure 17) five days after clinical treatment. Complete restoration of airiness in both lungs.

The given example allows us to visually compare the dynamics of the X-ray pattern in this observation with similar information that was presented above in Section 2.5. Illustrations 4 and 5, which were presented in the second chapter, are also a typical example, but only of the initial stage of our work. At that time, great importance was attached to intravenous infusions and replenishing the volume of circulating blood in the treatment of such patients. The last observation refers already to the period of work when infusion therapy, which became prohibited in the initial period of the disease, was replaced by first aid methods that can eliminate the causes of increasing circulatory disorders.

Materials on the role and significance of infusion therapy in the dynamics of the course of AP were presented above in the relevant sections. Unfortunately, currently, infusion therapy in severe patients with AP continues to be considered worldwide as an important and mandatory means of medical care in the practice of inpatient treatment. In this regard, it is necessary to pay attention once again to the fact that this therapeutic procedure has a stimulating effect on the development of the inflammatory process in the lung and its inclusion, especially in the initial period of the disease, can bring the opposite effect to the desired.

In the last example, it is necessary to pay attention to one more important feature. In this case (as in the entire group of similar observations), no attempts were made to identify the pathogen, and antibacterial therapy was a very primitive set of drugs that at that time already had characteristics with very questionable effectiveness. Nevertheless, the overall result clearly shows that the problematic quality of antibacterial therapy did not prevent the achievement of rapid success.

Every specialist reading these lines can compare the examples presented here with the materials of those patients who have been and are being treated in their clinic. The general statistics of inpatient treatment of AP, which is reflected in numerous publications on this topic, suggests that a more frequent example of modern coincidences will be cases when, against the background of intensive treatment, there is a tendency to negative dynamics of clinical and radiological signs.

On the other hand, achieving a rapid therapeutic effect, which corresponds to the last of our examples, is not a stable and permanent result in modern medicine. If someone can demonstrate such a result today, then it is unlikely that such a result refers to an observation with an aggressive development of the process, and such cases are the exception rather than the rule.

If we avoid criticizing the system of views on the essence of the AP, then we can discuss this problem endlessly, but without visible results. Inconsistencies between the concept of disease and fundamental science are becoming more and more noticeable every year, but there remains an unwillingness to see and perceive such contradictions. Current research and discussions on the problem of AP are focused on the micromechanisms of the process, while visual and tangible control over its dynamics gives way to various laboratory tests and virtual assessments. The current coverage of this disease in the professional literature shows that most specialists avoid touching on the basics of this topic, continuing to focus on theoretical stereotypes received at the university.

Recent events have shown that, despite the absolutely obvious change in the etiology of AP, not only have there been no fundamental changes in medical prescriptions, but, most importantly, this has not affected the essence of views on this problem. The appearance of a large number of patients with COVID-19 pneumonia during the SARS-CoV-2 pandemic did not significantly change either the theory of the disease or the practice of its treatment.

On the one hand, the unshakable belief in the leading role of the pathogen remained the same and even intensified, thanks to the peculiarities of transmission of the virus. Although, as attention was drawn to this feature above, the transmission of the pathogen and the very fact of the development of the disease are not identical concepts.

On the other hand, viral lung tissue damage, in which the previous principles of treatment based on the leading role of antibiotics have lost even their theoretical significance, continue to be stubbornly used in general practice. The nature of treatment, conditioned by the ideology of the disease and determining its results, continues to adhere to the previous models of medical care, in which antibiotics retain their leading place among medical prescriptions for COVID-19 pneumonia worldwide (107-116,331).

Various attempts to find criteria for differential diagnosis between CAP and COVID-19 pneumonia ultimately proved unsuccessful (117,118,161,444,445). At the same time, the absence of convincing differences between bacterial and viral forms of inflammation in the lung tissue is another proof that the nature of the pathogen is not of fundamental importance for clinical, radiological and laboratory signs of the process, and we are talking about the same disease in the light of the basic canons of medicine. However, this undoubted fact remains unnoticed, since scientific research and practical solutions in this area continue to be determined by the role of the pathogen as the main cause of all the troubles that arise.

During the SARS-CoV-2 pandemic, the problem in the treatment of patients with coronavirus pneumonia was clearly manifested. Today it has already become obvious that the vast majority of infected people who have signs of the disease overcome this event on their own, without special medical care. However, when the disease progresses and hospitalization is required, modern medicine can offer nothing but symptomatic and supportive care. The average mortality rate among hospitalized patients with COVID-19 pneumonia worldwide is 21%, while in Asian countries it is 13%, in the USA it is 20%, in Europe it is 23% and reaches 30% in South America (446).

The figures presented do not mean at all that the quality of official medicine in the countries of the Asian region is significantly higher than in the United States or in Europe. Treatment of patients with AP is carried out in accordance with a single standard worldwide without significant differences between continents and countries, and therefore various statistical indicators cannot depend on nuances in treatment approaches. In order to understand the essence of the problem in such a critical situation and find its solution, it is necessary, first of all, to go beyond the existing system of views and re-analyze current events from the point of view of the general laws of nature and medical science. However, the existing ideas about the problem of AP have been formed, remembered and practiced for many years, defining the boundaries of permissible diagnostic and therapeutic actions.

Since the formation of general ideas about the nature of AP took place under the symbol of antibiotics, the importance of the microbiology of the process continues to support the previous strategy when searching for solutions in a new situation. In this regard, interest in the study of nosocomial infections began to grow again. For example, during such an analysis, it was noted that coronavirus infection among those hospitalized in hospitals can reach 41% (447), and mortality in hospital infection is higher than in the case of infection at home (448).

Previously, with bacterial forms of AP, the cause of higher mortality among patients in the hospital was explained by their infection after hospitalization with a more virulent microflora. No one has provided reasoned and objective evidence about this, although the reason for the higher mortality in such patients is quite understandable and does not directly depend on the type of pathogen of AP. If a patient already has health problems and against this background he gets pneumonia, then it will be much more difficult for him to overcome this catastrophe than for a healthy person who has the disease against the background of complete well-being, right? The same reasons determine the difference in the final results among patients with COVID-19 pneumonia.

To understand these statistics correctly, it should be remembered that healthy people are not placed in a hospital, and hospitalization is usually used in patients in emergency cases or with certain deviations in the state of the body, in which it is impossible to provide outpatient care. The presence of such patients in the same building with coronavirus carriers for quite a long time and at a relatively close distance significantly increases the risk of their infection, and then they turn into the most severe contingent. In the end, these circumstances served as a logical reason for the organization of specialized departments for patients with SARS-CoV-2.

The experience of organizing specialized departments for patients with COVID-19 pneumonia has shown that this measure has not changed the overall picture of the final results, but the former ghosts of the fatal role of nosocomial infection remain one of the working options for search directions. Such studies are continuing in the midst of the SARS-CoV-2 pandemic against bacterial strains, and their results, which show that such bacterial infection can reach 49%, encourage the use of antibiotics (7,449,450). However, the reliability and significance of these statistics, from my point of view, are a reflection of previous illusions, and, in addition to the reason for the preservation of antibiotics among the means of treating patients with coronavirus, they further reinforce misconceptions, making it difficult to understand the basics of AP.

The last remarks are based on those well-known and actually generally recognized facts that the accuracy and reliability of methods for determining the pathogens of AP cause more questions than they give the necessary answers. In addition, in order to claim that infection with certain strains of bacteria occurred after hospitalization within the walls of the hospital, it is necessary, at least, to have similar comparative results of microbiological analyses on the eve of hospitalization, isn't it? It was not possible to find such comparative studies in the available literature, and the isolation of so-called nosocomial pneumonia was an attempt to improve the choice of antibiotics and increase the effectiveness of treatment, but this initiative remained at the level of clinical assumptions, without bringing noticeable practical success in previous years.

Currently, the direction and content of the ongoing research reflect the efforts and attempts of medical science to create a universal remedy for pneumonia. But while the results of such a search remain at the level of intentions, the definition of risk factors and criteria for predicting mortality from this disease continues in parallel (209, 451-454). At the same time, forecasts of fatal outcomes are developed for a period of at least 30 days, which is the best indicator of the uncertainty that exists in relation to modern AP treatment.

The announcement of the appearance of an active drug against coronavirus was supposed to give confidence to those who are waiting for a "pill for pneumonia". However, the results of testing of molnupiravir showed that this drug, with early use, can only slightly reduce the risk of possible hospitalization and mortality, leaving the whole problem in the same state of expected solutions (455).

In conditions of constant dynamics of etiological factors, the dreams of developing etiotropic drugs, as well as other proposals to improve the effectiveness of medical care for these patients, are frankly "cosmetic" in nature. For example, it has been statistically established that oxygen supply to severe patients with AP in the prone positioning for 6 hours a day reduces the risk of their intubation, and for 8 hours slightly reduces mortality (456). But after all, this technique does not contribute to immediate recovery, does not eliminate the existing danger of developing critical conditions and does not lead to a significant improvement in overall treatment indicators, does it?

Or, for example, at the height of the pandemic, when hospitals around the world are filled mainly with patients with COVID-19 pneumonia, pneumococcus is presented as one of the main causative agents of CAP and attention is drawn to the decrease in the effectiveness of anti-pneumococcal vaccines with the justification of increasing their polyvalence (56-58). Such information looks more like it was prepared at the request of a party interested in increasing the production of such drugs than the logical requirement of the current situation. This looks all the more strange if we return to the results of pneumococcal vaccination of the population, when this type of pathogen significantly exceeded its current percentage in the etiology of AP. As noted above, a slight decrease in morbidity after the start of vaccination did not lead to a noticeable decrease in mortality, and the number of complicated forms of the disease even increased.

As the current situation shows, attempts to solve the AP problem by preserving the old strategy in the new conditions of the pandemic have not brought any noticeable success over a period of more than 2 years and have not added confidence in the work of medical care systems. Moreover, there is a further deepening of already existing misconceptions, especially in the group of the most severe patients with viral pneumonia. In this cohort of patients, the problem of AP is closely intertwined with the problem of sepsis due to general ideas about the mechanisms of disease development. Such a convergence of two urgent problems as a result of a distortion of views on the pathogenesis of pulmonary localization of inflammation gives incorrect statistics of septic complications.

It makes sense to take another look at the problem of septic complications in AP, which most clearly reflects modern misconceptions in helping patients with acute inflammatory processes of the bronchopulmonary system. To date, sepsis is one of the leading causes of morbidity and mortality, which, according to world statistics, accounts for 50 million cases annually, of which 11 million are fatal, which is 20% of all deaths in the world (457). In the United States, sepsis accounts for 1.7 million cases of medical treatment every year, and it is the main cause of hospital mortality (458-460).

In the general group of cases of sepsis, the most common cause of its development is considered to be CAP, which accounts for up to half of the cases of this complication (25,336-338). In turn, when analyzing the clinical materials of patients hospitalized with CAP in hospitals, in 30 percent or more of such cases, the disease proceeds with the development of sepsis and septic shock (25,339). Despite such impressive statistics of the dominant development of septic complications among patients with inflammation of the lung tissue, it was this category of patients that attracted attention when, in the vast majority of cases, the pathogen was not detected in the blood during examination (104,105). The explanation was usually the previous use of antibiotics, which for some reason did not affect bacteriological studies in other diseases.

To the non-standard features of sepsis in patients with AP, it is necessary to add such facts from observations of recent years as further deterioration of the condition of patients after hospitalization already against the background of ongoing treatment with the development of septic complications that were absent at admission, the lack of significance of early antibacterial therapy for the dynamics of the disease, an increase in the number of pleural complications up to 50 percent or more already within the walls of hospitals, an increase in mortality rates, which, according to some statistics, losses reflect every second patient, transferred to the intensive care unit (24,25,83,85,130,158,167,172,173,198,244-246,266,270,326,443,461-463).

Analyzing the results of treatment of sepsis and septic shock, F. Cavelli et al. (324) note that, despite the expansion of our knowledge about these conditions, they are still difficult to treat, and mortality remains high. A more categorical conclusion was made by K.E. Rudd et al. (457), who argue that, despite the huge financial costs of studying sepsis, there are no effective methods of its treatment, except awareness of it and the use of antibiotics.

If, according to the latter opinion, antibiotics are considered as the only group of drugs for the treatment of sepsis, then the comparative results of their earliest possible use do not give any advantages (308-311,331,464), which does not allow their effect to be considered decisive in the outcome of the disease. As for awareness of these septic complications, in this case, the authors unwittingly noted the reason on which further decisions depend, and we returned to the issue that we have already discussed above. That is, in this case, the accuracy and validity of the diagnosis of septic complications should be discussed.

The materials of modern research and clinical trials on the problem of AP allow us to note one very common feature. Many reports on such work clearly show that the authors, when starting to implement it, already see in advance the result that should be obtained. And since the expected result does not always come at the finish line, very often the conclusions end with a standard recommendation that the effect is not achieved, but these studies need to be continued. At the same time, as noted above, the answer to the question posed may not always confirm our assumptions, and the results obtained may suggest the right direction of the search.

For many recent years, there has been an intensified fight against sepsis, the frequency of which among hospitalized patients with AP reaches 30 percent or more, and one of its cardinal signs is considered to be a violation of peripheral, not pulmonary hemodynamics. At the same time, such confirmation of sepsis as the presence of bacteremia usually does not exceed 10%. Usually, such statistics include patients without a complicated course of the disease in this indicator. In the light of such information, the question should logically arise as to whether sepsis in general is such a common cause of the severe condition of patients with AP? But no one attaches importance to the specifics of the localization of AP and the specifics of functional disorders of the affected organ, and the decision-making strategy in this group of patients continues on the basis of analogies with other inflammatory processes.

Today, these analogies dictate the principles of treatment of patients with COVID-19 pneumonia, when its most severe manifestations also begin to be explained by sepsis, but only of viral etiology. Unlike bacterial variants of septic complications, in the latter group there is no objective evidence that the cause of sepsis and septic shock is a virus, and diagnostic criteria for these conditions are automatically taken from the general settings for all inflammatory processes (85,86, 104, 105, 125-129,131,132). Attempts at differential diagnosis of bacterial and viral variants of the disease, not to mention more detailed differences depending on the pathogen, were unsuccessful, but this "lesson" remained misunderstood.

The futility of attempts to distinguish the AP variant depending on its pathogen shows the fallacy of this direction, since the observed clinical features are due to other factors. Regardless of the constantly occurring changes among the nonspecific pathogens of inflammatory processes in the lung tissue, we are still talking about one nosological form, which equally includes CAP, nosocomial pneumonia, viral lesions and other varieties that appeared under the banner of the leading role of microbiological factors in their origin.

Having created stereotypes of providing medical care to patients with AP, based on general assessments and interpretations of the whole variety of acute inflammatory diseases, modern medicine reaps the fruits of its own simplified generalizations. Nature contrasted the purpose of the lungs in the general circulatory system with all other organs and tissues of the body. When, under the conditions of such preliminary circumstances, a standard correction of deviations resulting from inflammation is carried out, the results of such correction will depend on the localization of the primary focus. This is an axiom, the scientific foundations of which have been discovered and proven by medical science, which now does not attach due importance to them in practical implementation.

Analysis of the results of AP treatment over the past decades shows a slow but steady decline in the effectiveness of medical care for this category of patients. In addition to medical statistics, which were presented in the course of this presentation quite widely and in various ways, it is necessary to note the economic side of this process. Evaluation and discussion of the costs of treatment of patients with CAP showed a constant increase in this indicator (465,466). A few years ago, it was noted that, for example, in the United States, the total annual cost of treating patients with CAP has increased from $10.6 billion to $17 billion in recent years, with 90% of this amount allocated to inpatient treatment (467,468).

The figures presented are further evidence that the principles of providing medical care to patients with AP need a radical revision. The growing costs of implementing the maximum possible, from a modern point of view, medical support mainly go to the inpatient, the most difficult stage of medical care, but these financial injections do not save the situation, and the lethality and the number of complications of AP, at best, remain stable, although in fact they continue to grow.

Bringing the AP ideology in line with the canons of medical science and further changing approaches to treatment in general practice is a long overdue necessity. This process is inevitable, but it cannot have an easy and short path. It takes time and continuous hard work before you can see and evaluate the first successes. Today, the discrepancy between the fundamentals of medical science and the scientific representation of the problem of AP has become much more noticeable and obvious than four decades ago, when the concentration of the most severe cases of the disease forced us to take the first steps in search of an optimal solution.

The links and materials presented here, if necessary, can be found among the publications in order to get acquainted with their content in more detail and conduct additional analysis of them. But, the main feature of the information presented here is that it is presented from a point of view that does not correspond to generally accepted ideas about the problem under discussion and even contradicts them. In this situation, specific conclusions can be perceived as an attempt to offer unambiguous and indisputable recommendations, which was not part of the plans for writing this manuscript. You can change your point of view on the problem only as a result of your own checks and conclusions.

As already noted above, the presented work is, first of all, information for reflection. In order for such an analysis not to be only theoretical, it is reasonable, without changing anything, to check the effectiveness of the treatment principles used today not by statistical comparisons of results in different groups of observations, but to find objective criteria for the therapeutic effect of various methods of care. At the same time, it is very important not only to find objective assessment methods, but also to obtain visual confirmation that a particular therapeutic method affects the patient's condition. For example, if as a result of treatment there are shifts at the cellular and molecular levels, then this fact is not yet proof that the patient has become easier, right?

The last wishes concern, first of all, the methods of primary medical care. If the majority of patients with AP do not need hospitalization yet and overcome the disease mainly on their own, then with the aggressive development of the process, their future fate is determined by the nature and pathogenetic direction of the first emergency care. That is why adequate counteraction to the dynamics of inflammation should be a priority and as early as possible in the treatment of AP.

The only conclusion that states the facts is that by now there has been a distorted idea of the nature of acute inflammatory processes of the lung tissue. The materials presented above are indisputable evidence of the formation of a *destructive meme* in this section of medicine (469,470). The interpretation of the essence of the affected problem in full dependence on the properties of the pathogen was formed under the influence of an excessively hypertrophied role of antibiotics in the treatment of this category of patients. The psychological and mental influence of this ideology determines the biased and limited search for a solution to the problem, which continues to replicate it, despite changing conditions. Correcting the dissonance in the existing concept of the disease is the inevitable and most difficult step, on which further results depend.

BIBLIOGRAPHY

1. World Health Organization. The top 10 causes of death. May 2018 [internet publication].
2. D.B. Hornick (2019). Community-Acquired Pneumonia Update 2019. https://familyphysician.centerforconferences.uiowa.edu/sites/familyphysician.centerforconferences.uiowa.edu/files/hornick_douglas_-_pneumonia_update.pdf
3. Ahmad FB, Cisewski JA, Miniño A, Anderson RN. (2021). Provisional Mortality Data — United States, 2020. MMWR Morb Mortal Wkly Rep 2021; 70:519–522. DOI: http://dx.doi.org/10.15585/mmwr.mm7014e1external icon
4. Alimi Y, Lim WS, Lansbury L, et al. (2017). Systematic review of respiratory viral pathogens identified in adults with community-acquired pneumonia in Europe. J Clin Virol. 2017 Oct;95:26-35.
5. WHO. Global Health Estimates: Life expectancy and leading causes of death and disability. (2021). https://www.who.int/data/gho/data/themes/mortality-and-global-health-estimates
6. J. P. Metlay, G. W. Waterer, A. C. Long at al.; on behalf of the American Thoracic Society and Infectious Diseases Society of America (2019). "Diagnosis and Treatment of Adults with Community-acquired Pneumonia. An Official Clinical Practice Guideline of the American Thoracic Society and Infectious Diseases Society of America". American Journal of Respiratory and Critical Care Medicine, Volume 200, Issue 7, 1 October 2019, Pages e45-e67, https://www.atsjournals.org/doi/full/10.1164/rccm.201908-1581ST
7. Puzniak, L., Finelli, L., Yu, K.C. et al. (2021). A multicenter analysis of the clinical microbiology and antimicrobial usage in hospitalized patients in the US with or without COVID-19. BMC Infect Dis 21, 227 (2021). https://doi.org/10.1186/s12879-021-05877-3
8. Pulia, M., Wolf, I., Schwei, R., Chen, D., Lepak, A., Schulz, L., & Safdar, N. (2021). Antibiotic prescribing patterns for coronavirus

disease 2019 (COVID-19) in two emergency departments with rapid procalcitonin. Infection Control & Hospital Epidemiology, 42(3), 359-361. doi:10.1017/ice.2020.1329

9. Montes-Andujar L, Tinoco E, Baez-Pravia O, et al. (2021). Empiric antibiotics for community-acquired pneumonia in adult patients: a systematic review and a network meta-analysis. Thorax Published Online First: 15 March 2021. doi: 10.1136/thoraxjnl-2019-214054
10. Alejandro David Bendala Estrada, Jorge Calderón Calderón Parra, Eduardo Fernández Carracedo et al. (2021). Inadequate Use of Antibiotics in the Covid-19 Era: Effectiveness of Antibiotic Therapy, 01 March 2021, PREPRINT (Version 1) available at Research Square [https://doi.org/10.21203/rs.3.rs-244297/v1]
11. Rudan I, Boschi-Pinto C, Biloglav Z, Mulholland K, Campbell H. Epidemiology and etiology of childhood pneumonia. Bull World Health Organ. 2008; 86:408–416. [PMC free article] [PubMed] [Google Scholar]
12. WHO Revised global burden of disease 2002 estimates. 2004. http://www.who.int/healthinfo/global_burden_disease/estimates_regional_2002_revised/en/ (accessed Nov 5, 2010).
13. Ruuskanen O, Lahti E, Jennings LC, Murdoch DR (April 2011). "Viral pneumonia". Lancet. 377 (9773): 1264–75. doi:10.1016/S0140-6736(10)61459-6.
14. https://en.wikipedia.org/wiki/Severe_acute_respiratory_syndrome
15. Paula Peyrani, Lionel Mandell, Antoni Torres & Glenn S Tillotson (2019) The burden of community-acquired bacterial pneumonia in the era of antibiotic resistance, Expert Review of Respiratory Medicine, 13:2, 139-152, DOI: 10.1080/17476348.2019.1562339
16. Attaway A H, Scheraga R G, Bhimraj A (2021). Severe covid-19 pneumonia: pathogenesis and clinical management. BMJ, 2021; 372 :n436 doi:10.1136/bmj.n436
17. Ing AJ, Cocks C, Green JP (2020). COVID-19: in the footsteps of Ernest Shackleton. Thorax, 2020;75:693-694.
18. Z. Wu, J. M. McGoogan (2020). Characteristics of and Important Lessons From the Coronavirus Disease 2019 (COVID-19) Outbreak in China. Summary of a Report of 72 314 Cases From the Chinese Center for Disease Control and Prevention. JAMA. 2020;323(13): 1239-1242. doi:10.1001/jama.2020.2648

19. Merad, M., Martin, J.C. Pathological inflammation in patients with COVID-19: a key role for monocytes and macrophages. Nat Rev Immunol 20, 355–362 (2020). https://doi.org/10.1038/s41577-020-0331-4
20. Ra SH, Lim JS, Kim G, et al. (2021). Upper respiratory viral load in asymptomatic individuals and mildly symptomatic patients with SARS-CoV-2 infection. Thorax, 2021;76:61-63.
21. A. Liapikou, E. Rosales-Mayor, A. Torres (2014). The management of severe community acquired pneumonia in the ICU. June 2014, Expert Review of Respiratory Medicine 8(3): 293-303.DOI: 10.1586/17476348.2014.896202
22. J. W. Kim, J.J. Kim, H. J. Yang at al.(2015). The Prognostic Factors of Pneumonia with Septic Shock in Patients Presenting to the Emergency Department. Korean Journal of Critical Care Medicine 2015; 30(4): 258-264
23. P. Jason, N. C. Dean, Q. Guo et al. (2016). Severe community-acquired pneumonia: timely management measures in the first 24 hours. Critical Care,2016,20:237
24. A. Vidal, L. Santos (2017). Comorbidities impact on the prognosis of severe acute community-acquired pneumonia. Porto Biomedical Journal, Vol. 2. Num. 6. November - December 2017, pages 247-346
25. A. Ceccato, A. Torres (2018). Sepsis and community-acquired pneumonia. Ann Res Hosp 2018; 2:7
26. Grasselli G et al. (2020). Baseline characteristics and outcomes of 1591 patients infected with SARS-CoV-2 admitted to ICUs of the Lombardy region, Italy. JAMA 2020 Apr 6; [e-pub]. (https://doi.org/10.1001/jama.2020.5394)
27. S. Richardson, J. S. Hirsch, M. Narasimhan at al. (2020). Presenting Characteristics, Comorbidities, and Outcomes Among 5700 Patients Hospitalized With COVID-19 in the New York City Area. JAMA. Published online April 22, 2020. doi:10.1001/jama.2020.6775
28. Renato Seligman and Beatriz Graeff Santos Seligman (2020). "Pandemic in the 21st Century. The Challenge of COVID-19". EC Pulmonology and Respiratory Medicine 9.8 (2020): 30-31.
29. Gupta S, Wang W, Hayek SS, et al. Association between early treatment with tocilizumab and mortality among critically ill patients with COVID-19. JAMA Intern Med. 2020;180(11):1436-1446. doi:10.1001/jamainternmed.2020.3596

30. Lai J, Ma S, Wang Y, et al. (2020). Factors associated with mental health outcomes among health care workers exposed to coronavirus disease 2019. JAMA Netw Open 2020;3(3):e203976-e203976.
31. R. E. Leiter (2020). Reentry. NEJM, October 14, 2020. DOI: 10.1056/NEJMp2027447
32. J. N. Rosenquist (2020). The Stress of Bayesian Medicine — Uncomfortable Uncertainty in the Face of Covid-19. NEJM, N Engl J Med 2021; 384:7-9. DOI: 10.1056/NEJMp2018857
33. Xu Chen. "Avoiding Defensive Medicine among Pandemic". EC Emergency Medicine and Critical Care 4.12 (2020): 49-53.
34. Kader, N., Elhusein, B., Chandrappa, N.S.K. et al. (2021). Perceived stress and post-*traumatic* stress disorder symptoms among intensive care unit staff caring for severely ill coronavirus disease 2019 patients during the pandemic: a national study. Ann Gen Psychiatry 20, 38 (2021). https://doi.org/10.1186/s12991-021-00363-1
35. Matteo Nioi, Pietro Emanuele Napoli, Jessica Lobina et al. (2021). COVID-19 and Italian Healthcare Workers From the Initial Sacrifice to the mRNA Vaccine: Pandemic Chrono-History, Epidemiological Data, Ethical Dilemmas, and Future Challenges. Front. Public Health, 21 January 2021. https://doi.org/10.3389/fpubh.2020.591900
36. Erdem H., Lucey D.R. (2021). Healthcare worker infections and deaths due to COVID-19: a survey from 37 nations and a call for WHO to post national data on their website. Int J Infect Dis. 2021; 102: 239-241
37. WHO Solidarity Trial Consortium (2020). Repurposed Antiviral Drugs for Covid-19 — Interim WHO Solidarity Trial Results. February 11, 2021, N Engl J Med 2021; 384:497-511. DOI: 10.1056/NEJM oa 2023184
38. Mo Shehata (2020). "Covid-19; The Possible Medical Strategies". EC Pulmonology and Respiratory Medicine 9.6 (2020): 03-07.
39. D. A. Berlin, R. M. Gulick, F. J. Martinez (2020). Severe Covid-19. December 17, 2020. N Engl J Med 2020; 383:2451-2460. DOI: 10.1056/NEJMcp2009575
40. Mayank Vats., et al.(2020). "Second Wave of COVID-19 - Could it be More Lethal!!! - Novel 6 T's Strategies May Help". EC Pulmonology and Respiratory Medicine 9.8 (2020): 17-21.

41. Amr Abdel-Mordy Kandeel (2020). Do We Need Changes in Management Strategies of COVID-19 Pandemic? Vitamin D as a Balance Key for Health-Economy Dilemma. http://dx.doi.org/10.5281/zenodo.3782752, Iberoam J Med, vol.2, n4, p.250-252, 2020
42. V. E. Schaye, J. A. Reich, B. P. Bosworth et al. (2020). Collaborating Across Private, Public, Community, and Federal Hospital Systems: Lessons Learned from the Covid-19 Pandemic Response in NYC. NEJM Catalyst Innovations in Care Delivery 2020; 06, Vol. 1 No. 6, November — December 2020. DOI:https://doi.org/10.1056/CAT.20.0343
43. V. J. Dzau, C. Balatbat (2020). Strategy, coordinated implementation, and sustainable financing needed for COVID-19 innovations. The Lancet Journal, Nov 07, 2020, Volume 396, Number 10261p1463-1534, e73-e82.
44. El-Shimy, IA, Mohamed, MM, Hasan, SS, Hadi, MA. (2021). Targeting host cell proteases as a potential treatment strategy to limit the spread of SARS-CoV-2 in the respiratory tract. Pharmacol Res Perspect. 2021; 9:e00698. https://doi.org/10.1002/prp2.698
45. Feigin R (2004). Textbook of Pediatric Infectious Diseases (5th ed.). Philadelphia: W. B. Saunders. p. 299. ISBN 978-0-7216-9329-3.
46. Bloodletting. https://en.wikipedia.org/wiki/Bloodletting#Further_reading
47. George Washington. https://en.wikipedia.org/wiki/George_Washington
48. Leech. https://en.wikipedia.org/wiki/Leech
49. Cupping therapy. https://en.wikipedia.org/wiki/Cupping_therapy
50. Ice bath. https://en.wikipedia.org/wiki/Ice_bath
51. Whole body cryotherapy. In: Cryotherapy. https://en.wikipedia.org/wiki/Cryotherapy#Whole_body_cryotherapy
52. Versporten A, Zarb P, Caniaux I, Gros MF, Drapier N, Miller M, et al. (2018). Antimicrobial consumption and resistance in adult hospital inpatients in 53 countries: results of an internet-based global point prevalence survey. Lancet Glob Health. 2018;6(6):e619–29.
53. Plotkin, Stanley; Orenstein, W; Offit, PA (September 22, 2012). Vaccines. Elsevier – Saunders. p. 542. ISBN 978-1455700905. Retrieved July 2, 2015.

54. F.Tokgoz Akyil,,M.Yalcinsoy A.Hazar,,A.Cilli B.Celenk O.Kilic A.Sayiner N.KokturkfA.Sakar Coskun A.Filiz E.Cakir Edis (2018). "iPrognosis of hospitalized patients with community-acquired pneumonia". Pulmonology. Volume 24, Issue 3, May–June 2018, Pages 164-169
55. Pletz MW, Rohde GG, Welte T et al. (2016). Advances in the prevention, management, and treatment of community-acquired pneumonia [version 1; referees: 2 approved]. F1000Research 2016, 5(F1000 Faculty Rev):300 (doi: 10.12688/f1000research.7657.1)
56. Pick H, Daniel P, Rodrigo C, et al . Pneumococcal serotype trends, surveillance and risk factors in UK adult pneumonia, 2013-18. Thorax 2020;75:37–48.
57. Goldblatt D, Miller E. Editorial. Pneumococcal pneumonia. Thorax 2020;75-1
58. R. Isturiz, L. Grant, S. Gray et al. (2021). Expanded Analysis of 20 Pneumococcal Serotypes Associated With Radiographically Confirmed Community-Acquired Pneumonia in Hospitalized US Adults, Clinical Infectious Diseases, 2021; ciab375, https://doi.org/10.1093/cid/ciab375
59. Jain S, Self WH, Wunderink RG et al. (2015). Community- Acquired Pneumonia Requiring Hospitalization among U.S. Adults. N Engl J Med. 2015;373(5):415. Epub 2015 Jul 14.
60. C. Castillo (2020). 2020 IDCA/ATS Community-Acquired Pneumonia Guideline: more micro, less macrolide, no HCAP. 15th Annual NW Regional Hospital Medicine Conference. September 25, 2020
61. https://www.cdc.gov/mrsa/community/#community
62. Aliberti S, Zanaboni AM, Wiemken T, Nahas A, Uppatla S, Morlacchi LC, Ramirez J. (2012). Criteria for clinical stability in hospitalised patients with community-acquired pneumonia. European Respiratory Journal. 2012; 42(3): 742–749. doi:10.1183/09031936.00100812
63. Mohammad, A.K., Nasir, M., Paul, S., Rahman, H., Abul, K. and Ahmed, F.U. (2020). Common Pathogens and Their Resistance to Antimicrobials in Community Acquired Pneumonia (CAP): A Single Center Study in Bangladesh. International Journal of Medical Science and Clinical Invention. 7, 12 (Dec. 2020), 5144–5153. DOI:https://doi.org/10.18535/ijmsci/v7i12.04.
64. Pneumonia-Wikipedia. https://en.wikipedia.org/wiki/Pneumonia

65. Li, S.T., Tancredi, D.J. (2010). Empyema Hospitalizations Increased in US Children Despite Pneumococcal Conjugate Vaccine. Pediatrics. 2010: 125: 26-33. Ref.: https://goo.gl/aPX2JW
66. Strachan RE, Snelling TL, Jaffé A (2013). Increased paediatric hospitalizations for empyema in Australia after introduction of the 7-valent pneumococcal conjugate vaccine. Bull World Health Organ. 2013; 91: 167-173. Ref.: https://goo.gl/MXTYqQ
67. Wuerth, B. A., Bonnewell, J. P., Wiemken, T. L., & Arnold, F. W. (2016). Trends in Pneumonia Mortality Rates and Hospitalizations by Organism, United States, 2002–2011. Emerging Infectious Diseases, 22(9), 1624-1627. https://doi.org/10.3201/eid2209.1506
68. Pneumococcal vaccine. https://en.wikipedia.org/wiki/Pneumococcal_vaccine
69. Pneumococcal polysaccharide vaccine https://en.wikipedia.org/wiki/Pneumococcal_polysaccharide_vaccine
70. Arnold D, Hamilton F, Morris T, et al. (2019). S12 The changes in incidence and management of pleural empyema in England over the last decade. Thorax, 2019;74: A9-A10.
71. Bobbio A, Bouam S, Frenkiel J, et al. (2021). Epidemiology and prognostic factors of pleural empyema. Thorax, Published Online First: 30 March 2021. doi: 10.1136/thoraxjnl-2020-215267
72. B. Bannister, S. Gillespie, J. Jones. Infection: microbiology and management. Published by Blackwell Publishing Ltd, Blackwell Publishing, Inc., 350 Main Street, Malden, Massachusetts 02148-5020, USA, Third edition 2006, ISBN-13: 978-1-4051-2665-6
73. Pneumonia. World Health Organization. https://www.who.int/news-room/fact-sheets/detail/pneumonia
74. Davis CP. (1996). Normal Flora. In: Baron S, editor. Medical Microbiology. 4th edition. Galveston (TX): University of Texas Medical Branch at Galveston; 1996. Chapter 6. Available from: https://www.ncbi.nlm.nih.gov/books/NBK7617/
75. https://en.wikipedia.org/wiki/Streptococcus_pneumoniae#Biotechnology
76. Garcia-Vidal C, Ardanuy C, Tubau F, et al. Pneumococcal pneumonia presenting with septic shock: host- and pathogen-related factors and outcomes. Thorax 2010; 65:77-81.
77. Salvà-Serra, Francisco; Connolly, Gwendolyn; Moore, Edward R. B.; Gonzales-Siles, Lucia (2017-12-15). "Detection of "Xisco" gene for

identification of Streptococcus pneumoniae isolates". Diagnostic Microbiology and Infectious Disease. 90 (4): 248–250. doi:10.1016/j.diagmicrobio.2017.12.003. ISSN 1879-0070. PMID 29329755.

78. https://www.cdc.gov/pneumonia/epic/index.html
79. Sharma S, Maycher B, Eschun G (May 2007). "Radiological imaging in pneumonia: recent innovations". Current Opinion in Pulmonary Medicine. 13 (3): 159–69.
80. Igor Klepikov (2019). Concepts and reliability of the etiology of acute pneumonia. Hong Kong Journal of Peadiatric Research. 2019;2(1):01-04
81. Klepikov I. (2020). How many pneumonias exist in nature? Eur J Clin Microbiol Infect Dis (2020). https://doi.org/10.1007/s10096-020-03834-7
82. Alhazzani W et al. (2020). Surviving sepsis campaign: Guidelines on the management of critically ill adults with coronavirus disease 2019 (COVID-19). Crit Care Med 2020 Mar 27; [e-pub]. (https://doi.org/10.1097/CCM.0000000000004363)
83. L. J. Schlapbach, N. Kissoon, A. Alhawsawi et al. (2020). World Sepsis Day: a global agenda to target a leading cause of morbidity and mortality. August 2020, AJP Lung Cellular and Molecular Physiology, 319(3). DOI: 10.1152/ajplung.00369.2020
84. Prescott HC, Girard TD. (2020). Recovery From Severe COVID-19: Leveraging the Lessons of Survival From Sepsis. JAMA. 2020; 324(8):739–740. doi:10.1001/jama.2020.14103
85. Singer M, Deutschman CS, et al. (February 2016). "The Third International Consensus Definitions for Sepsis and Septic Shock (Sepsis-3)". JAMA. 315 (8): 801–10. doi:10.1001/jama.2016.0287. PMC 4968574. PMID 26903338.
86. Rhodes A, Evans LE, et al. (March 2017). "Surviving Sepsis Campaign: International Guidelines for Management of Sepsis and Septic Shock: 2016". Intensive Care Medicine. 43 (3): 304–377. doi:10.1007/s00134-017-4683-6. PMID 28101605.
87. G. W. Waterer, M. W. Quasney, R. M. Cantor, R. G. Wunderink (2001). Septic Shock and Respiratory Failure in Community-acquired Pneumonia Have Different TNF Polymorphism Associations. AJRCCM,Vol.163,No 7,Jun 01,2001 https://doi.org/10.1164/ajrccm.163.7.2011088

88. Sanjay Sethi (2020). Community-Acquired Pneumonia. Merck Manual for the Professional. https://www.merckmanuals.com/professional

89. Hadil A.AlOtair, Mohammed A.Hussein, Mohamed A.Elhoseny et al. (2015). Severe pneumonia requiring ICU admission: Revisited. Journal of Taibah University Medical Sciences. Volume 10, Issue 3, September 2015, Pages 293-299. https://doi.org/10.1016/j.jtumed.2015.03.005

90. Inflammation. https://en.wikipedia.org/wiki/Inflammation

91. Schwiegk, H. (1935). Der Lungenentlastungsreflex. Pflügers Arch. ges. Physiol. 236, 206–219 (1935).

92. Klepikov I (2017). The Meaning of Pulmonary Reflexes in the Pathogenesis of Acute Pneumonia. Intern Med 7:232. doi: 10.4172/2165-8048.1000232

93. Thillai M, Patvardhan C, Swietlik EM, et al. (2021). Functional respiratory imaging identifies redistribution of pulmonary blood flow in patients with COVID-19. Thorax 2021; 76:182-184.

94. Renin–angiotensin system https://en.wikipedia.org/wiki/Renin%E2%80%93angiotensin_system

95. Pulmonary embolism. https://en.wikipedia.org/wiki/Pulmonary_embolism

96. Elliott C G. (1992). Pulmonary physiology during pulmonary embolism Chest 1992,101(4, Suppl):163S–171S. [PubMed] [Google Scholar]

97. Lualdi JC, Goldhaber SZ (1995). "Right ventricular dysfunction after acute pulmonary embolism: pathophysiologic factors, detection, and therapeutic implications". Am Heart J. 130 (6): 1276–82. PMID 7484782.

98. Smulders Y M. Pathophysiology and treatment of haemodynamic instability in acute pulmonary embolism: the pivotal role of pulmonary vasoconstriction. Cardiovasc Res. 2000;48(01):23–33. [PubMed] [Google Scholar]

99. Turetz M, Sideris AT, Friedman OA, Triphathi N, Horowitz JM. Epidemiology, Pathophysiology, and Natural History of Pulmonary Embolism. Semin Intervent Radiol. 2018;35(2):92–98. doi:10.1055/s-0038-1642036

100. Goldhaber SZ (2005). "Pulmonary thromboembolism". In Kasper DL, Braunwald E, Fauci AS, et al. (eds.). Harrison's Principles of Internal

Medicine (16th ed.). New York: McGraw-Hill. pp. 1561–65. ISBN 978-0-07-139140-5.

101. Blood pressure. https://en.wikipedia.org/wiki/Blood_pressure#Pulmonary_pressure

102. Liapikou A, Ferrer M, Polverino E et al. (2009). Severe Community-Acquired Pneumonia: Validation of the Infectious Diseases Society of America/American Thoracic Society Guidelines to Predict an Intensive Care Unit Admission. Clin Infect Dis 2009; 48: 377–85. pmid:19140759

103. Restrepo MI, Mortensen EM, Rello J et al. (2010). Late admission to the ICU in patients with community-acquired pneumonia is associated with higher mortality. Chest, 2010; 137: 552–57. pmid:19880910

104. Lin GL, McGinley JP, Drysdale SB et al (2018). Epidemiology and immune pathogenesis of viral sepsis. Front Immunol, 9:2147

105. Weiss, S.L., Peters, M.J., Alhazzani, W. et al. (2020). Surviving sepsis campaign international guidelines for the management of septic shock and sepsis-associated organ dysfunction in children. Intensive Care Med 46, 10–67 (2020). https://doi.org/10.1007/s00134-019-05878-6

106. Aliberti S, Zanaboni AM, Wiemken T, Nahas A, Uppatla S, Morlacchi LC, Ramirez J.(2012). Criteria for clinical stability in hospitalised patients with community-acquired pneumonia. European Respiratory Journal. 2012; 42(3): 742–749. doi:10.1183/09031936.00100812

107. J. A. Jernigan, K. M. Hatfield, H. Wolford et al. (2020). Multidrug-Resistant Bacterial Infections in U.S. Hospitalized Patients, 2012–2017.N Engl J Med 2020; 382:1309-1319. DOI: 10.1056/NEJMoa1914433

108. Montes-Andujar L, Tinoco E, Baez-Pravia O, et al. (2021). Empiric antibiotics for community-acquired pneumonia in adult patients: a systematic review and a network meta-analysis. Thorax 2021;76: 1020-1031.

109. Rawson TM, Moore LSP, Zhu N, et al. (2020). Bacterial and fungal co-infection in individuals with coronavirus: A rapid review to support COVID-19 antimicrobial prescribing [published online ahead of print, 2020 May 2]. Clin Infect Dis. 2020; ciaa 530. doi:10.1093/cid/ciaa530

110. B. O'Kelly, C. Cronin, D. Connellan et al. (2021). Antibiotic prescribing patterns in patients hospitalized with COVID-19: lessons from the first wave, JAC-Antimicrobial Resistance, Volume 3, Issue 2, June 2021, dlab085, https://doi.org/10.1093/jacamr/dlab085

111. Puzniak, L., Finelli, L., Yu, K.C. et al. (2021). A multicenter analysis of the clinical microbiology and antimicrobial usage in hospitalized patients in the US with or without COVID-19. BMC Infect Dis 21, 227 (2021). https://doi.org/10.1186/s12879-021-05877-3

112. Kim D, Quinn J, Pinsky B et al. (2020). Rates of co-infection between SARS-CoV-2 and other respiratory pathogens. JAMA 2020; 323: 2085–6.

113. B.Beović, M. Doušak, J. Ferreira-Coimbra et al. (2020). Antibiotic use in patients with COVID-19: a 'snapshot' Infectious Diseases International Research Initiative (ID-IRI) survey. Journal of Antimicrobial Chemotherapy, dkaa326, https://doi.org/10.1093/jac/dkaa326

114. Ocampo-Torres Moisés., et al. (2020). "Characterization of Mortality by Covid-19 in a Health System in Central Mexico". EC Pulmonology and Respiratory Medicine 9.12 (2020): 20-22

115. Alejandro David Bendala Estrada, Jorge Calderón Calderón Parra, Eduardo Fernández Carracedo et al. (2021). Inadequate Use of Antibiotics in the Covid-19 Era: Effectiveness of Antibiotic Therapy, 01 March 2021, PREPRINT (Version 1) available at Research Square [https://doi.org/10.21203/rs.3.rs-244297/v1]

116. B.D. Huttner,G. Catho,J.R. Pano-Pardo et al. (2020). COVID-19: don't neglect antimicrobial stewardship principles! Clinical Microbiology and Infection, Vol 26, Issue 7, P808-810. Published:April 29, 2020, DOI:https://doi.org/10.1016/j.cmi.2020.04.024

117. C. Heneghan, A. Pluddemann, K. R. Mahtani (2020). Differentiating viral from bacterial pneumonia. April 8, 2020. The Centre for Evidence-Based Medicine. Evidence Service to support the COVID-19 response. University of Oxford. https://www.cebm.net/covid-19/differentiating-viral-from-bacterial-pneumonia.

118. Lipman M, Chambers RC, Singer M, et al. (2020). SARS-CoV-2 pandemic: clinical picture of COVID-19 and implications for research. Thorax 2020; 75:614-616.

119. Revised WHO classification and treatment of childhood pneumonia at health facilities. Geneva: World Health Organization, 2014.

120. A-S. Ginsburg, T. Mvalo, E. Nkwopara et al. (2020). Amoxicillin for 3 or 5 Days for Chest-Indrawing Pneumonia in Malawian Children. N Engl J Med 2020; 383:13-23. DOI: 10.1056/NE
121. A. B. Chang, K. Grimwood (2020). Antibiotics for Childhood Pneumonia — Do We Really Know How Long to Treat? July 2, 2020, N Engl J Med 2020; 383:77-79 DOI: 10.1056/NEJMe2016328
122. WHO Solidarity Trial Consortium (2020). Repurposed Antiviral Drugs for Covid-19 — Interim WHO Solidarity Trial Results. February 11, 2021, N Engl J Med 2021; 384:497-511. DOI: 10.1056/NEJM oa 2023184
123. Azithromycin. https://en.wikipedia.org/wiki/Azithromycin
124. Gyselinck I, Janssens W, Verhamme P, et al. (2021). Rationale for azithromycin in COVID-19: an overview of existing evidence. BMJ, Open Respiratory Research 2021;8:e000806. doi: 10.1136/bmjresp-2020-000806
125. Lim TK, Chew MY. (2018). Management of severe community acquired pneumonia in the emergency department. J Emerg Crit Care Med 2018;2:2.
126. Knaus WA, Draper EA, Wagner DP, Zimmerman JE. (1985). APACHE II: a severity of disease classification system. Crit Care Med. 1985 Oct;13(10):818-29. PMID: 3928249.
127. Murillo-Zamora, E, Medina-Gonzalez, A, Zamora-Perez, L, et al. (2018) Performance of the PSI and CURB-65 scoring systems in predicting 30-day mortality in healthcare-associated pneumonia. Med Clin (Barc) 150: 99–103.
128. Ilg, A, Moskowitz, A, Konanki, V, et al. (2019) Performance of the CURB-65 score in predicting critical care interventions in patients admitted with community-acquired pneumonia. Ann Emerg Med 74: 60–68.
129. Junnian Chen, Bang Liu, Houwei Du et al. (2021). Performance of CURB-65, PSI, and APACHE-II for predicting COVID-19 pneumonia severity and mortality. European Journal of Inflammation, Volume 19, 2021, https://doi.org/10.1177/20587392211027083
130. Hassan, M., Patel, S., Sadaka, A. S., Bedawi, E. O., Corcoran, J. P., & Porcel, J. M. (2021). Recent Insights into the Management of Pleural Infection. International journal of general medicine, 14, 3415–3429. https://doi.org/10.2147/IJGM.S292705
131. WHO. Clinical management of severe acute respiratory infection (SARI) when COVID-19 disease is suspected. Interim guidance 13

March 2020. https://www.who.int/docs/default-source/coronaviruse/clinical-management-of-novel-cov.pdf

132. CDC. Interim Clinical Guidance for Management of Patients with Confirmed Coronavirus Disease (COVID-19). Updated Feb. 16, 2021. https://www.cdc.gov/coronavirus/2019-ncov/hcp/clinical-guidance-management-patients.html
133. Roger C. (2021). COVID-19: should we consider it as a septic shock? (The treatment of COVID-19 patients in the ICU). Curr Opin Anaesthesiol. 2021 Apr 1;34(2):119-124. doi: 10.1097/ACO.0000000000000956. PMID: 33470663.
134. Hajjar LA, Costa IBSDS, Rizk SI, Biselli B. et al. (2021). Intensive care management of patients with COVID-19: a practical approach. Ann Intensive Care. 2021 Feb 18;11(1):36. doi: 10.1186/s13613-021-00820-w. PMID: 33604873; PMCID: PMC7891474.
135. Klepikov I. (1989). “Acute pneumonia and its purulent and destructive complications in children in the midst of a major industrial centre of Western Siberia”. Dissertation for the degree of doctor of medical sciences. Leningrad (1989).
136. Lung microbiota. https://en.wikipedia.org/wiki/Lung_microbiota
137. Sachs L. "Statistische Auswertungsmethoden". Springer Verlag. Berlin, Heidelberg, New York, 1972
138. Allergy. https://en.wikipedia.org/wiki/Allergy
139. Menkin Valy. “Dinamics of inflammation”. Macmillan (1940).
140. Klepikov I., Rikov V. (1990) "The way to design synpneumonias pleurisy"- Author's certificate for invention, SU, No 1631574, A1,1 november 1990, USSR
141. Lobar pneumonia. https://en.wikipedia.org/wiki/Lobar_pneumonia
142. Cotran R.S.; Kumar V.; Fausto N.; at al.; (2005). Robbins and Cotran pathologic basis of disease. St. Louis, Mo: Elsevier Saunders. p. 749. ISBN 0-7216-0187-1.
143. M.A. Elemraid, M.F. Thomas, A.P. Blain at al. Risk Factors for the Development of Pleural Empyema in Children. Pediatric Pulmonology 50:721–726 (2015)
144. Patria, M. F., Longhi, B., Lelii, M. at al. (2013). Association between radiological findings and severity of community-acquired pneumonia in children. Italian journal of pediatrics, 39, 56. https://doi.org/10.1186/1824-7288-39-56
145. http://www.cdc.gov/media/releases/2015/p0225-pneumonia-

hospitalizations.html

146. J. Gafford et al. (2021). "The Vanderbilt Open-Source Ventilator: From Napkin Sketch to Ready to Save Lives in Three Weeks," in IEEE Robotics & Automation Magazine, vol. 28, no. 1, pp. 101-114, March 2021, doi: 10.1109/MRA.2020.3045668.
147. Rice TW, Janz DR. (2020). In Defense of Evidence-based Medicine for the Treatment of COVID-19 Acute Respiratory Distress Syndrome. Ann Am Thorac Soc. 2020 Jul;17(7):787-789. doi: 10.1513/AnnalsATS.202004-325IP. PMID: 32320268; PMCID: PMC7328187.
148. Truog RD, Mitchell C, Daley GQ. (2020). The toughest triage — allocating ventilators in a pandemic. N Engl J Med 2020; 382:1973-1975.
149. J. H. Stone, M. J. Frigault, N. J. Serling-Boyd et al. (2020). Efficacy of Tocilizumab in Patients Hospitalized with Covid-19. NEJM, October 21, 2020, DOI: 10.1056/NEJMoa2028836
150. M. Ackermann, S. E. Verleden, M. Kuehnel at al. (2020). Pulmonary Vascular Endothelialitis, Thrombosis, and Angiogenesis in Covid-19. May 21, 2020. DOI: 10.1056/NEJMoa2015432
151. Martines RB, Ritter JM, Matkovic E et al; COVID-19 Pathology Working Group (2020). Pathology and Pathogenesis of SARS-CoV-2 Associated with Fatal Coronavirus Disease, United States. Emerg Infect Dis. 2020 Sep;26(9):2005-2015. doi: 10.3201/eid2609.202095. Epub 2020 May 21. PMID: 32437316; PMCID: PMC7454055.
152. Doctrine. https://en.wikipedia.org/wiki/Doctrine
153. Zhou, B, Kojima, S, Kawamoto, A, Fukushima, M. COVID-19 pathogenesis, prognostic factors, and treatment strategy: Urgent recommendations. J Med Virol. 2021; 1– 11. https://doi.org/10.1002/jmv.26754
154. Chandrasoma P, Taylor CR (2005). "Part A. "General Pathology", Section II. "The Host Response to Injury", Chapter 3. "The Acute Inflammatory Response", sub-section "Cardinal Clinical Signs"". Concise Pathology (3rd ed.). McGraw-Hill. ISBN 978-0-8385-1499-3. OCLC 150148447. Retrieved 5 November 2008.
155. Raimondi GA. (2003). Intercambio gaseoso en el síndrome de dificultad respiratoria aguda [Gas exchange in acute respiratory distress syndrome]. Medicina (B Aires). 2003;63(2):157-64. Spanish. PMID: 12793087.

156. Radermacher P, Maggiore SM, Mercat A. (2017). Fifty years of research in ARDS: gas exchange in acute respiratory distress syndrome. Am J Respir Crit Care Med 2017; 196:964–984.
157. Hepokoski, M. L., Odish, M., & Malhotra, A. (2018). Prone positioning in acute respiratory distress syndrome: why aren't we using it more?. Journal of thoracic disease, 10(Suppl 9), S1020–S1024. https://doi.org/10.21037/jtd.2018.04.60
158. Gattinoni L, Gattarello S, Steinberg I, et al. (2021). COVID-19 pneumonia: pathophysiology and management. Eur Respir Rev 2021; 30: 210138 [DOI: 10.1183/16000617.0138-2021].
159. P. Haouzi, A. Zamir, E. Villarreal-Fernandez et al. (2020). Mechanics of Breathing and Gas Exchange in Mechanically Ventilated Patients with COVID-19–associated Respiratory Failure. American Journal of Respiratory and Critical Care Medicine, Volume 202, Issue 4 https://doi.org/10.1164/rccm.202004-1041LE
160. E. Barbeta, A. Motos, A. Torres et al. (2020). SARS-CoV-2–induced Acute Respiratory Distress Syndrome: Pulmonary Mechanics and Gas-Exchange Abnormalities. Annals of the American Thoracic Society, Volume 17, Issue 9
https://doi.org/10.1513/AnnalsATS.202005-462RL
161. S-Y Ruan, C-T Huang, Y-C Chien et al. (2021). Etiology-associated heterogeneity in acute respiratory distress syndrome: a retrospective cohort study. BMC Pulm Med (2021) 21:183
https://doi.org/10.1186/s12890-021-01557-9
162. Olivia Vynn (2001). Cardiology secrets. Chapter 41, p. 210. Adair Edition: 2, illustrated Published by Elsevier Health Sciences, 2001 ISBN 1-56053-420-6, 978-1-56053-420-4,
163. Klepikov I. (2018). Acute Pneumonia is More Cardiovascular than Respiratory Disaster. J Emerg Med Care 1(1):105
164. Multiple organ dysfunction syndrome.
https://en.wikipedia.org/wiki/Multiple_organ_dysfunction_syndrome
165. Irwin, Richard S.; Rippe, James M. (2003). Irwin and Rippe's Intensive Care Medicine. Lippincott Williams & Wilkins. ISBN 978-0-7817-3548-3
166. Vincent JL, Moreno R, Takala J, et al. (1996). The SOFA (Sepsis-related Organ Failure Assessment) score to describe organ dysfunction/failure. On behalf of the Working Group on Sepsis-

Related Problems of the European Society of Intensive Care Medicine. Intensive Care Med 1996;22:707-10. [Crossref] [PubMed]

167. Reid PT, and Innes, JA. (2018). Respiratory Medicine. In: Ralston, SH, Penman ID, Strachan MWJ, Hobson RP (eds) Davidson's principles and practice of Medicine. 23rd ed. 2018; China: Churchill Livingstone Elsevier, pp.583-585.
168. Rollas K, Ersan G, Zincircioğlu et al. (2021). Septic shock in patients admitted to intensive care unit with COVID-19 pneumonia. Eurasian J Pulmonol 2021;23:95-100
169. Systemic inflammatory response syndrome. https://en.wikipedia.org/wiki/Systemic_inflammatory_response_syndrome
170. "American College of Chest Physicians/Society of Critical Care Medicine Consensus Conference: definitions for sepsis and organ failure and guidelines for the use of innovative therapies in sepsis" (1992). Crit. Care Med. 20 (6): 864–74. 1992. doi:10.1097/00003246-199206000-00025. PMID 1597042. S2CID 20057097.
171. Levy MM, Fink MP, Marshall JC, Abraham E, Angus D, Cook D, Cohen J, Opal SM, Vincent JL, Ramsay G (Apr 2003). "2001 SCCM/ ESICM/ACCP/ATS/SIS International Sepsis Definitions Conference". Crit Care Med. 31 (4): 1250–1256. doi:10.1097/01.CCM.0000050454.01978.3B. PMID 12682500. S2CID 19605781.
172. Prina E, Ranzani OT, Torres A (September 2015). "Community-acquired pneumonia". Lancet. 386 (9998): 1097–108. doi:10.1016/S0140-6736(15)60733-4. PMC 7173092. PMID 26277247.
173. Phua J, Dean NC, Guo Q, Kuan WS, Lim HF, Lim TK (August 2016). "Severe community-acquired pneumonia: timely management measures in the first 24 hours". Critical Care. 20 (1): 237. doi:10.1186/s13054-016-1414-2. PMC 5002335. PMID 27567896.
174. Pfeifer M, Hamer OW. (2020). COVID-19-Pneumonie [COVID-19 pneumonia]. Internist (Berl). 2020 Aug;61(8):793-803. German. doi: 10.1007/s00108-020-00854-5. PMID: 32728817; PMCID: PMC7388437.
175. Akbar Mohammadrezaei (2021). "Covid-19 Treatment from a New Perspective for the First Time". Acta Scientific Microbiology 5.3 (2021): 62-65.

176. Cytokine. https://en.wikipedia.org/wiki/Cytokine
177. Cytokine storm. https://en.wikipedia.org/wiki/Cytokine_storm
178. D. C. Fajgenbaum, C. H. June (2020). Cytokine Storm. N Engl J Med 2020; 383:2255-2273. DOI: 10.1056/NEJMra2026131
179. Ye, Q., Wang, B., & Mao, J. (2020). The pathogenesis and treatment of the `Cytokine Storm' in COVID-19. The Journal of infection, 80(6), 607–613. https://doi.org/10.1016/j.jinf.2020.03.037
180. Tang, Y., Liu, J., Zhang, D., Xu, Z., Ji, J., & Wen, C. (2020). Cytokine Storm in COVID-19: The Current Evidence and Treatment Strategies. Frontiers in immunology, 11, 1708. https://doi.org/10.3389/fimmu.2020.01708
181. Panigrahy, D., Gilligan, M. M., Huang, S., Gartung, A., Cortés-Puch, I., Sime, P. J., Phipps, R. P., Serhan, C. N., & Hammock, B. D. (2020). Inflammation resolution: a dual-pronged approach to averting cytokine storms in COVID-19?. Cancer metastasis reviews, 39(2), 337–340. https://doi.org/10.1007/s10555-020-09889-4
182. Farah H, et al. (2020). Potential Anti-Inflammatory Approaches for the Management of SARS-CoV2 Infections. J Pulmon Respir Sci 2020, 5(S1): 000S1-001.
183. Cytokine Storm -to the Editor. (2021). April 22, 2021. N Engl J Med 2021; 384:e59. DOI: 10.1056/NEJMc2036236
184. Caramaschi, S., Kapp, M.E., Miller, S.E. et al. (2021). Histopathological findings and clinicopathologic correlation in COVID-19: a systematic review. Mod Pathol (2021). https://doi.org/10.1038/s41379-021-00814-w
185. Hyperthermia. https://en.wikipedia.org/wiki/Hyperthermia#Personal_protective_equipment
186. "Hyperthermia to Treat Cancer" (2021). National Cancer Institute. https://www.cancer.gov/about-cancer/treatment/types/hyperthermia
187. Wiese, O. J., Allwood, B. W., & Zemlin, A. E. (2020). COVID-19 and the renin-angiotensin system (RAS): A spark that sets the forest alight? Medical hypotheses, 144, 110231. https://doi.org/10.1016/j.mehy.2020.110231
188. Saavedra JM. (2020). Angiotensin receptor blockers and COVID-19. Pharmacol Res. 2020 Jun;156:104832. doi: 10.1016/j.phrs.2020.104832. Epub 2020 Apr 15. PMID: 32304747; PMCID: PMC7158830.

189. Aleksova A, Ferro F, Gagno G, Cappelletto C, Santon D, Rossi M, Ippolito G, Zumla A, Beltrami AP, Sinagra G. (2020). COVID-19 and renin-angiotensin system inhibition: role of angiotensin converting enzyme 2 (ACE2) - Is there any scientific evidence for controversy? J Intern Med. 2020 Oct;288(4):410-421. doi: 10.1111/joim.13101. Epub 2020 Jun 8. PMID: 32459372; PMCID: PMC7283873.
190. Sanchis-Gomar, F., Lavie, C. J., Perez-Quilis, C., Henry, B. M., & Lippi, G. (2020). Angiotensin-Converting Enzyme 2 and Antihypertensives (Angiotensin Receptor Blockers and Angiotensin-Converting Enzyme Inhibitors) in Coronavirus Disease 2019. Mayo Clinic proceedings, 95(6), 1222–1230. https://doi.org/10.1016/j.mayocp.2020.03.026
191. D. Clark Files, Kevin W. Gibbs, Christopher L. Schaich et al. (2021). A Pilot Study to Assess the Circulating Renin-Angiotensin-System in COVID-19 Acute Respiratory Failure. American Journal of Physiology-Lung Cellular and Molecular Physiology. 19 MAY 2021, https://doi.org/10.1152/ajplung.00129.2021
192. Christiansen CF, Pottegård A, Heide-Jørgensen U, et al. (2021). SARS-CoV-2 infection and adverse outcomes in users of ACE inhibitors and angiotensin-receptor blockers: a nationwide case-control and cohort analysis. Thorax 2021;76:370-379.
193. Felsenstein S, Herbert JA, McNamara PS, Hedrich CM. (2020). COVID-19: Immunology and treatment options. Clin Immunol. 2020 Jun;215:108448. doi: 10.1016/j.clim.2020.108448. Epub 2020 Apr 27. PMID: 32353634; PMCID: PMC7185015.
194. NIH. COVID-19 Treatment Guidelines. https://www.covid19treatmentguidelines.nih.gov/therapies/immunomodulators/summary-recommendations/
195. Alijotas-Reig, J., Esteve-Valverde, E., Belizna, C., Selva-O'Callaghan, A., Pardos-Gea, J., Quintana, A., Mekinian, A., Anunciacion-Llunell, A., & Miró-Mur, F. (2020). Immunomodulatory therapy for the management of severe COVID-19. Beyond the anti-viral therapy: A comprehensive review. Autoimmunity reviews, 19(7), 102569. https://doi.org/10.1016/j.autrev.2020.102569
196. Sattui, S. E., Crow, M. K., & Navarro-Millán, I. (2021). The role of immunomodulatory medications in the treatment of COVID-19. Current opinion in rheumatology, 33(5), 431–445. https://doi.org/10.1097/BOR.0000000000000817

197. Rizk JG, Kalantar-Zadeh K, Mehra MR, Lavie CJ, Rizk Y, Forthal DN. (2020). Pharmaco-Immunomodulatory Therapy in COVID-19. Drugs. 2020 Sep;80(13):1267-1292. doi: 10.1007/s40265-020-01367-z. PMID: 32696108; PMCID: PMC7372203.

198. Abeldaño Zuñiga RA, Coca SM, Abeldaño GF, González-Villoria RAM. (2021). Clinical effectiveness of drugs in hospitalized patients with COVID-19: a systematic review and meta-analysis. Ther Adv Respir Dis. 2021 Jan-Dec;15:17534666211007214. doi: 10.1177/17534666211007214. PMID: 33765902; PMCID: PMC8010807.

199. W.Alhazzani,M.Alshahrani,F.Alshamsi et al. (2021). The Saudi Critical Care Society practice guidelines on the management of COVID-19 in the ICU: therapy section. Journal of Infection and Public Health. https://doi.org/10.1016/j.jiph.2021.10.005 Available online 20 October 2021

200. C. Grimm, S. Dickel, J. Grundmann et al. (2021). Case Report: Interferon-γ Rescues Monocytic Human Leukocyte Antigen Receptor (mHLA-DR) Function in a COVID-19 Patient With ARDS and Superinfection With Multiple MDR 4MRGN Bacterial Strains. October 2021, Frontiers in Immunology, 12:753849 DOI: 10.3389/fimmu.2021.753849

201. Kory P, Kanne JP (2020). SARS-CoV-2 organising pneumonia: 'Has there been a widespread failure to identify and treat this prevalent condition in COVID-19? BMJ, Open Respiratory Research, 2020;7:e000724. doi: 10.1136/bmjresp-2020-000724

202. Vadász I, Husain-Syed F, Dorfmüller P, et al. (2020). Severe organising pneumonia following COVID-19. Thorax. Published Online First: 11 November 2020. doi: 10.1136/thoraxjnl-2020-216088

203. Ahmed I. Siddiqi., (2020) Cytokine flames of COVID-19. J. Archives of Medical Case Reports and Case Study. 3(2); DOI:10.31579/2692-9392/014

204. H. Clifford Lane and Anthony S. Fauci (2021). Research in the Context of a Pandemic. N Engl J Med 2021; 384:755-757. DOI: 10.1056/NEJMe2024638

205. The RECOVERY Collaborative Group (2021). Dexamethasone in Hospitalized Patients with Covid-19. N Engl J Med 2021; 384:693-704. DOI: 10.1056/NEJMoa2021436

206. Abeldaño Zuñiga RA, Coca SM, Abeldaño GF et al. (2021). Clinical effectiveness of drugs in hospitalized patients with COVID-19: a systematic review and meta-analysis. Ther Adv Respir Dis. 2021 Jan-Dec; 15:17534666211007214. doi: 10.1177/17534666211007214. PMID: 33765902; PMCID: PMC8010807.
207. Andrew J. McArdle, Ortensia Vito, Harshita Patel et al. (2021). Treatment of Multisystem Inflammatory Syndrome in Children. N Engl J Med 2021; 385:11-22. DOI: 10.1056/NEJMoa2102968
208. Mary Beth F. Son, Nancy Murray, Kevin Friedman et al. (2021). Multisystem Inflammatory Syndrome in Children — Initial Therapy and Outcomes. N Engl J Med 2021; 385:23-34. DOI: 10.1056/NEJMoa2102605
209. Singh AP, Shady A, Gbaje E, et al. (2021). Factors associated with survival in patients with COVID -19 admitted to a community hospital in New York City. J Lung Pulm Respir Res. 2021;8(2):27–33. DOI: 10.15406 /jlprr.2021.08.00247
210. Fan DM (2017). Integrative medicine: Theory and practice [m]. World Book Publishing Company, China.
211. Jun M. (2021). Clinical Study on Prevention, Treatment and Health Management of 2019-nCoV Pneumonia in China. 2021- 3(6) OAJBS.ID.000275. DOI: 10.38125/OAJBS.000275
212. Pneumonia with a negative chest x-ray: Clinical diagnoses, physician documentation, and coding guidelines. JustCoding News: Inpatient, December 7, 2011. http://www.hcpro.com/content.cfm?dp=HIM&content_id=273998
213. M. S. Niederman (2018). Imaging for the Management of Community-Acquired Pneumonia. What to Do if the Chest Radiograph Is Clear. Chest, Editorial, Volume 153, Issue 3, P. 583-585, March 01, 2018
214. Seo H, Cha SI, Shin KM, Lim JK, Yoo SS, Lee SY, Lee J, Kim CH, Park JY. (2019). Community-Acquired Pneumonia with Negative Chest Radiography Findings: Clinical and Radiological Features. Respiration. 2019;97(6):508-517. doi: 10.1159/000495068. Epub 2019 Jan 9. PMID: 30625485.
215. Hunton R. (2019). Updated concepts in the diagnosis and management of community-acquired pneumonia. JAAPA. 2019 Oct;32(10):18-23. doi: 10.1097/01.JAA.0000580528.33851.0c. PMID: 31513034.

216. A. S. Brett (2018). Pneumonia with Negative Chest X-Ray but Positive CT Scan. NEJM Journal Watch, General Medicine. https://www.jwatch.org/na46290/2018/03/08/pneumonia-with-negative-chest-x-ray-positive-ct-scan
217. Thomas, J., Pociute, A., Kevalas, R., Malinauskas, M., & Jankauskaite, L. (2020). Blood biomarkers differentiating viral versus bacterial pneumonia aetiology: a literature review. Italian journal of pediatrics, 46(1), 4. https://doi.org/10.1186/s13052-020-0770-3
218. Korppi M, Don M, Valent F, Canciani M. The value of clinical features in differentiating between viral, pneumococcal and atypical bacterial pneumonia in children. Acta Paediatr. 2008 Jul;97(7):943-7. doi: 10.1111/j.1651-2227.2008.00789.x. Epub 2008 Apr 15. PMID: 18422803.
219. Arshad SH, Tariq SM, Matthews S, Hakim E. (2001). Sensitization to common allergens and its association with allergic disorders at age 4 years: a whole population birth cohort study. Pediatrics. 2001 Aug;108(2):E33. doi: 10.1542/peds.108.2.e33. PMID: 11483843.
220. Platts-Mills TA, Erwin E, Heymann P, Woodfolk J (2005). "Is the hygiene hypothesis still a viable explanation for the increased prevalence of asthma?". Allergy. 60 Suppl 79: 25–31. doi:10.1111/j.1398-9995.2005.00854.x. PMID 15842230. S2CID 36479898.
221. Bloomfield SF, Stanwell-Smith R, Crevel RW, Pickup J (April 2006). "Too clean, or not too clean: the hygiene hypothesis and home hygiene". Clinical and Experimental Allergy. 36 (4): 402–25. doi:10.1111/j.1365-2222.2006.02463.x. PMC 1448690. PMID 16630145.
222. Katz, Y., Gutierrez-Castrellon, P., González, M.G. et al. (2014). A Comprehensive Review of Sensitization and Allergy to Soy-Based Products. Clinic Rev Allerg Immunol 46, 272–281 (2014). https://doi.org/10.1007/s12016-013-8404-9
223. van Ree, R., Hummelshøj, L., Plantinga, M., Poulsen, L. K., & Swindle, E. (2014). Allergic sensitization: host-immune factors. Clinical and translational allergy, 4(1), 12. https://doi.org/10.1186/2045-7022-4-12
224. Sio, Y.Y., Pang, S.L., Say, YH. et al. (2021). Sensitization to Airborne Fungal Allergens Associates with Asthma and Allergic Rhinitis

Presentation and Severity in the Singaporean/Malaysian Population. Mycopathologia 186, 583–588 (2021). https://doi.org/10.1007/s11046-021-00532-6
225. Smith KR, Samet JM, Romieu I, et al. (2000). Indoor air pollution in developing countries and acute lower respiratory infections in children. Thorax 2000;55:518-532.
226. F. Orazzo, L. Nespoli, K. Ito et al. (2009). Air Pollution, Aeroallergens, and Emergency Room Visits for Acute Respiratory Diseases and Gastroenteric Disorders among Young Children in Six Italian Cities. Environmental Health Perspectives, Vol. 117, No. 11. https://doi.org/10.1289/ehp.0900599
227. Manisalidis I, Stavropoulou E, Stavropoulos A, Bezirtzoglou E. (2020). Environmental and Health Impacts of Air Pollution: A Review. Front Public Health. 2020 Feb 20;8:14. doi: 10.3389/fpubh.2020.00014. PMID: 32154200; PMCID: PMC7044178.
228. Wu, Y., Zhan, Q., Zhao, Q. (2021). Long-term Air Pollution Exposure Impact on COVID-19 Morbidity in China. Aerosol Air Qual. Res. 21, 200143. https://doi.org/10.4209/aaqr.2020.07.0413
229. J. Grigg (2021). Air Pollution and Respiratory Infection: An Emerging and Troubling Association. American Journal of Respiratory and Critical Care Medicine, Volume 198, Issue 6. https://doi.org/10.1164/rccm.201804-0614ED
230. Croft, D.P., Burton, D.S., Nagel, D.J. et al. (2021). The effect of air pollution on the transcriptomics of the immune response to respiratory infection. Sci Rep 11, 19436 (2021). https://doi.org/10.1038/s41598-021-98729-8
231. Cook D.R. (1986). Non-Respiratory Functions of the Lung. In: Stanley T.H., Petty W.C. (eds) Anesthesiology 1986. Developments in Critical Care Medicine and Anesthesiology, vol 11. Springer, Dordrecht. https://doi.org/10.1007/978-94-009-4251-6_5
232. Chapter 10. Nonrespiratory functions of the lung. Levitzky M.G.(Ed.), (2013). Pulmonary Physiology, 8e . McGraw Hill. https://accessmedicine.mhmedical.com/content.aspx?bookid=575&sectionid=42512988
233. Deepak Joseph, Raju K Puttaswamy, Hari Krovvidi (2013). Non-respiratory functions of the lung, Continuing Education in Anaesthesia Critical Care & Pain, Volume 13, Issue 3, June 2013, Pages 98–102, https://doi.org/10.1093/bjaceaccp/mks060

234. Lung. https://en.wikipedia.org/wiki/Lung
235. Levy, MN; Pappano, AJ. (2007) Cardiovascular Physiology, Mosby Elsevier. 9th edition, pp.172.
236. Stanfield, CL; Germann, WJ. (2008). Principles of Human Physiology, Pearson Benjamin Cummings. 3rd edition, pp.430-431.
237. Baroreceptor. https://en.wikipedia.org/wiki/Baroreceptor#Low-pressure_baroreceptors
238. J.G. Roosenburg, H. Deenstra (1954). Bronchial-Pulmonary Vascular Shunts in Chronic Pulmonary Affections. Chest, | Vol. 26, Issue 6, P664-671, December 01, 1954 DOI:https://doi.org/10.1378/chest.26.6.664
239. Stanton, Bruce M.; Koeppen, Bruce A., eds. (2008). Berne & Levy physiology (6th ed.). Philadelphia: Mosby/Elsevier. pp. 418–422. ISBN 978-0-323-04582-7.
240. Moore, K (2018). Clinically oriented anatomy (8th ed.). pp. 333–339. ISBN 9781496347213.
241. Luo W, Yu H, Gou J et al. (2020). Clinical pathology of critical patient with novel coronavirus pneumonia (COVID-19). Pathology & Pathobiology 2020:2020020407.
242. Selvaraj V, Dapaah-Afriyie K. (2020). Lung cavitation due to COVID-19 pneumonia. BMJ Case Reports CP 2020;13:e237245.
243. Light RW. (2006). Parapneumonic effusions and empyema. Proc Am Thorac Soc. 2006;3(1):75-80. doi: 10.1513/pats.200510-113JH. PMID: 16493154.
244. S. A. Sahn (2007). Diagnosis and Management of Parapneumonic Effusions and Empyema, Clinical Infectious Diseases, Volume 45, Issue 11, 1 December 2007, Pages 1480–1486, https://doi.org/10.1086/522996
245. McCauley, L., & Dean, N. (2015). Pneumonia and empyema: causal, casual or unknown. Journal of thoracic disease, 7(6), 992–998. https://doi.org/10.3978/j.issn.2072-1439.2015.04.36
246. S. A. Helgeson, B. T. Hiroto, S. J. Billings et al. (2018). Which patients with a parapneumonic effusion need a chest tube? Cleveland Clinic Journal of Medicine August 2018, 85 (8) 609-611; DOI: https://doi.org/10.3949/ccjm.85a.17036
247. Cough reflex. https://en.wikipedia.org/wiki/Cough_reflex
248. F. D. McCool, (2006). Global Physiology and Pathophysiology of Cough. Chest, Vol. 129, Issue 1, 48S-53S, January 01, 2006 DOI: https://doi.org/10.1378/chest.129.1_suppl.48S

249. M. B. Beasley (2010). The Pathologist's Approach to Acute Lung Injury. Arch Pathol Lab Med. 2010;134:719–727
250. Nowicki, J., & Murray, M. T. (2020). Bronchitis and Pneumonia. Textbook of Natural Medicine, 1196–1201.e1. https://doi.org/10.1016/B978-0-323-43044-9.00155-2
251. Fengyun Wang, Bin Fang, LiXin Zhou et al. (2021). Severe 2019 novel coronavirus pneumonia may cause lung bullae and bronchiectasis: A case report and concise literature review. European Journal of Inflammation. Volume 19, 2021. https://doi.org/10.1177/20587392211029081
252. Jain V, Vashisht R, Yilmaz G, et al. (2021). Pneumonia Pathology. [Updated 2021 Aug 4]. In: StatPearls [Internet]. Treasure Island (FL): StatPearls Publishing; 2021 Jan-. Available from: https://www.ncbi.nlm.nih.gov/books/NBK526116
253. Kim C.E., Griffiths W.J., Taylor P.W. (2009). Components derived from Pelargonium stimulate macrophage killing of Mycobacterium species. J Appl Microbiol. 2009;106(4):1184–1193.
254. Kamin W., Maydannik V., Malek F.A. (2010). Efficacy and tolerability of EPs 7630 in children and adolescents with acute bronchitis—a randomized, double-blind, placebo-controlled multicenter trial with a herbal drug preparation from Pelargonium sidoides roots. Int J Clin Pharmacol Ther. 2010;48(3):184–191.
255. Michaelis M., Doerr H.W., Cinatl J., Jr. (2011). Investigation of the influence of EPs([R]) 7630, a herbal drug preparation from Pelargonium sidoides, on replication of a broad panel of respiratory viruses. Phytomedicine. 2011;18(5):384–386.
256. Careddu D., Pettenazzo A. (2018). Pelargonium sidoides extract EPs 7630: a review of its clinical efficacy and safety for treating acute respiratory tract infections in children. Int J General Med. 2018;11:91–98. PubMed PMID: 29563828.
257. Anand R, McAuley DF, Blackwood B, et al. (2020). Mucoactive agents for acute respiratory failure in the critically ill: a systematic review and meta-analysis. Thorax Published Online First: 08 June 2020. doi: 10.1136/thoraxjnl-2019-214355
258. Braman SS. (2006). Chronic cough due to acute bronchitis: ACCP evidence-based clinical practice guidelines. Chest. 2006;129(1 suppl):95S–103S.
259. Chang CC, Cheng AC, Chang AB. (2012). Over-the-counter (OTC) medications to reduce cough as an adjunct to antibiotics for acute

pneumonia in children and adults. Cochrane Database Syst Rev. 2012 Feb 15;(2):CD006088. doi: 10.1002/14651858.CD006088.pub3. Update in: Cochrane Database Syst Rev. 2014;(3):CD006088. PMID: 22336815.

260. Kinkade S, Long NA. (2016). Acute Bronchitis. Am Fam Physician. 2016 Oct 1;94(7):560-565. PMID: 27929206.

261. D. Kim, I. Song, D. Yoon et al. (2019). Pediatric Codeine Prescriptions in Outpatient and Inpatient Settings in Korea. The American Journal of Managed Care, August 2019, Volume 25, Issue 8

262. Bronchiolitis obliterans. https://en.wikipedia.org/wiki/Bronchiolitis_obliterans

263. Pneumonia (Simple English Wikipedia). https://simple.wikipedia.org/wiki/Pneumonia

264. Mandal AK, Thadepalli H, Mandal AK, Chettipally U. (1998). Outcome of primary empyema thoracis: therapeutic and microbiologic aspects. Ann Thorac Surg. 1998 Nov;66(5):1782-6. doi: 10.1016/s0003-4975(98)00601-8. PMID: 9875789.

265. Y. Shahin, J. Duffy, D. Beggs et al. (2010). Surgical management of primary empyema of the pleural cavity: outcome of 81 patients, Interactive CardioVascular and Thoracic Surgery, Volume 10, Issue 4, April 2010, Pages 565–567, https://doi.org/10.1510/icvts.2009.215004

266. Sundaralingam, A., Banka, R. & Rahman, N.M. (2021). Management of Pleural Infection. Pulm Ther 7, 59–74 (2021). https://doi.org/10.1007/s41030-020-00140-7

267. Gross I, Gordon O, Cohen-Cymberknoh M, et al. (2019). Giant lung cysts following necrotizing pneumonia: Resolution with conservative treatment. Pediatric Pulmonology. 2019 Jun;54(6): 901-906. DOI: 10.1002/ppul.24321.

268. Domej W, Wenisch C, Demel U, Tilz GP. (2003). Vom pneumonischen Infiltrat zum parapneumonischen Erguss--vom Erguss zum Pleuraempyem: Internistische Aspekte parapneumonischer Ergussbildung und des Pleuraempyems [From pneumonic infiltration to parapneumonic effusion--from effusion to pleural empyema: internal medicine aspects of parapneumonic effusion development and pleural empyema]. Wien Med Wochenschr. 2003;153(15-16):349-53. German. doi: 10.1007/s10354-003-0008-1. PMID: 13677257.

269. N.A. Maskell, C.W. Davies, A.J. Nunn, E.L. Hedley, F.V. Gleeson, R. Miller, et al. (2005). U.K. Controlled trial of intrapleural streptokinase for pleural infection.N Engl J Med, 352 (2005), pp. 865-874
270. K. R. Shen, A. Bribriesco, T. Crabtree et al. (2017). The American Association for Thoracic Surgery consensus guidelines for the management of empyema. The Journal of Thoracic and Cardiovascular Surgery, Volume 153, Issue 6, June 2017, Pages e129-e146 https://doi.org/10.1016/j.jtcvs.2017.01.030
271. Brutsche MH, Tassi GF, Györik S, Gökcimen M, Renard C, Marchetti GP, Tschopp JM. (2005). Treatment of sonographically stratified multiloculated thoracic empyema by medical thoracoscopy. Chest. 2005 Nov;128(5):3303-9. doi: 10.1378/chest.128.5.3303. PMID: 16304276.
272. Davies HE, Davies RJO, Davies CWH (2010). Management of pleural infection in adults: British Thoracic Society pleural disease guideline. 2010, Thorax 2010;65:ii 41-ii 53.
273. Carter E, Waldhausen J, Zhang W, Hoffman L, Redding G. (2010). Management of children with empyema: Pleural drainage is not always necessary. Pediatr Pulmonol. 2010 May;45(5):475-80. doi: 10.1002/ppul.21200. PMID: 20425855.
274. Klepikov I (2019). When Does a Patient with Acute Pneumonia Need a Surgeon? SM J Pediatr Surg 4: 2.
275. Moreno-Pérez D, Andrés Martín A, Tagarro García A, Escribano Montaner A, Figuerola Mulet J, García García JJ, Moreno-Galdó A, Rodrigo Gonzalo de Lliria C, Saavedra Lozano J. (2015). Neumonía adquirida en la comunidad: tratamiento de los casos complicados y en situaciones especiales. Documento de consenso de la Sociedad Española de Infectología Pediátrica (SEIP) y Sociedad Española de Neumología Pediátrica (SENP) [Community acquired pneumonia in children: Treatment of complicated cases and risk patients. Consensus statement by the Spanish Society of Paediatric Infectious Diseases (SEIP) and the Spanish Society of Paediatric Chest Diseases (SENP)]. An Pediatr (Barc). 2015 Sep;83(3):217.e1-11. Spanish. doi: 10.1016/j.anpedi.2014.12.002. Epub 2015 Jan 22. PMID: 25617977.
276. T. R. Semenkovich, M. A. Olsen, V. Puri et al. (2018). Current State of Empyema Management. The Annals of Thoracic Surgery, Vol 105, Issue 6, P1589-1596, JUNE 01, 2018. 2018 DOI:https://doi.org/10.1016/j.athoracsur.2018.02.027

277. Elsayed HH, Mostafa A, Fathy E, Diab HS, Nofal IM, AbdelHamid OA, El-Bawab HY, ElNori AA. (2018). Thoracoscopic management of early stages of empyema: is this the golden standard? J Vis Surg. 2018 May 29;4:114. doi: 10.21037/jovs.2018.05.18. PMID: 29963403; PMCID: PMC5994441.
278. Meyer Sauteur, P.M.; Burkhard, A.; Moehrlen, U.; Relly, C.; Kellenberger, C.; Ruoss, K.; Berger, C. (2019). Pleural Tap-Guided Antimicrobial Treatment for Pneumonia with Parapneumonic Effusion or Pleural Empyema in Children: A Single-Center Cohort Study. J. Clin. Med. 2019, 8, 698. https://doi.org/10.3390/jcm8050698
279. Anselmo Andrés-Martína, Amparo Escribano Montanerb? Joan FiguerolaMulet et al. (2020). Consensus document on community-acquired pneumonia in children. SENP-SEPAR-SEIPDocumento de consenso sobre la neumonía adquirida en la comunidad en los niños. SENP-SEPAR-SEIP. Archivos de Bronconeumología (English Edition). Volume 56, Issue 11, November 2020, Pages 725-741
280. A.Tessitore, M. Patella, M. Giuliani et al. (2021). Surgical treatment of pleural empyema in Coronavirus disease 19 patients: the Southern Switzerland experience, Interactive CardioVascular and Thoracic Surgery, Volume 32, Issue 3, March 2021, Pages 367–370, https://doi.org/10.1093/icvts/ivaa269
281. Barglik, R., Grabowski, A., Korlacki, W., Pasierbek, M., & Modrzyk, A. (2021). Pleural empyema in children - benefits of primary thoracoscopic treatment. Wideochirurgia i inne techniki maloinwazyjne = Videosurgery and other miniinvasive techniques, 16(1), 264–272. https://doi.org/10.5114/wiitm.2020.97443
282. Poole P. S., Stark H. E., Stark P. (2011). Necrotizing Pneumonia, Pulmonary Abscess, and Lung Gangrene: Multiple Pathways to Lung Parenchymal Destruction, Contemporary Diagnostic Radiology: June 30, 2011 - Volume 34 - Issue 13 - p 1-6 doi: 10.1097/ 01.CDR.0000399282.53274.e9
283. M. Schweigert, A. Dubecz, M. Beron, D. Ofner, H. J Stein (2013). Surgical therapy for necrotizing pneumonia and lung gangrene. Thorac Cardiovasc Surg. 2013 Oct;61(7):636-41. doi: 10.1055/s-0032-1311551. Epub 2012 Oct 3.
284. Masters, I., Isles, A.F. & Grimwood, K. (2017). Necrotizing pneumonia: an emerging problem in children?. Pneumonia 9, 11 (2017). https://doi.org/10.1186/s41479-017-0035-0

285. Borczuk, A.C., Salvatore, S.P., Seshan, S.V. et al. (2020). COVID-19 pulmonary pathology: a multi-institutional autopsy cohort from Italy and New York City. Mod Pathol 33, 2156–2168 (2020). https://doi.org/10.1038/s41379-020-00661-1
286. Loffi M, Regazzoni V, Sergio P, Martinelli E, Stifani I, Quinzani F, Robba D, Cotugno A, Dede M, Danzi GB. (2020). Spontaneous pneumomediastinum in COVID-19 pneumonia. Monaldi Arch Chest Dis. 2020 Sep 29;90(4). doi: 10.4081/monaldi.2020.1399. PMID: 32990690.
287. Romano, N., Fischetti, A., & Melani, E. F. (2020). Pneumomediastinum Related to Covid-19 Pneumonia. The American journal of the medical sciences, 360(6), e19–e20. https://doi.org/10.1016/j.amjms.2020.06.003
288. Hazariwala, V., Hadid, H., Kirsch, D. et al. (2020). Spontaneous pneumomediastinum, pneumopericardium, pneumothorax and subcutaneous emphysema in patients with COVID-19 pneumonia, a case report. J Cardiothorac Surg 15, 301 (2020). https://doi.org/10.1186/s13019-020-01308-7
289. Sun R, Liu H, Wang X. (2020). Mediastinal emphysema, giant bulla, and pneumothorax developed during the course of COVID-19 pneumonia. Korean J Radiol 2020;21:541–544.
290. Reindl S, Al-Wheibi S, Umlauf J, Girdauskas E, Raab S. (2021). Pneumomediastinum bei schwerer COVID-19-Erkrankung: eine Fallserie von acht Patienten [Pneumomediastinum in Severe COVID-19-disease: a Case Series of Eight Patients]. Zentralbl Chir. 2021 Dec;146(6):612-616. German. doi: 10.1055/a-1666-8551. Epub 2021 Dec 6. PMID: 34872115.
291. V. Nedelcu, D. S. Gologanu, V. Micu et al. (2021). Pneumomediastinum in patients with Covid-19 pneumonia - case series. European Respiratory Journal 2021 58: PA3483; DOI: 10.1183/13993003.congress-2021.PA3483
292. Hamman L. Spontaneous mediastinal emphysema. Bull Johns Hopkins Hosp 1939; 64:1-21.
293. Pascal's law. https://en.wikipedia.org/wiki/Pascal%27s_law
294. Mohan V, Tauseen RA. (2020). Spontaneous pneumomediastinum in COVID-19. BMJ Case Rep. 2020 May 25;13(5):e236519. doi: 10.1136/bcr-2020-236519. PMID: 32457032; PMCID: PMC7252963.
295. Kouritas VK, Papagiannopoulos K, Lazaridis G, et al. (2015). Pneumomediastinum. J Thorac Dis, 2015;7:S44–9.

296. Zhou C, Gao C, Xie Y, et al. (2020). COVID-19 with spontaneous pneumomediastinum. Lancet Infect Dis, 2020;20:510.
297. Campisi A, Poletti V, Ciarrocchi AP, et al. (2020). Tension pneumomediastinum in patients with COVID-19. Thorax 2020; 75:1130-1131.
298. I. Novakov, F. Shterev, S. Novakova (2021). Pneumomediastinum as a complication of COVID-19 pneumonia: a self-experience study. EMJ Respir. 2021;9[1]:57-58. Abstract Review No. AR4.
299. J. B. Romero, J. I. Hidalgo, E. M. Botejara et al. (2005). Spontaneous Pneumopericardium in a Patient With Community-Acquired Pneumonia. Revista Espanola de Cardiologia. Vol. 58. Issue 2.pages 227-229 (February 2005)
300. Roberto Scacciavillani, Giulia Iannaccone, Marco Giuseppe Del Buono, Giuseppe Bello (2020). Pneumopericardium following mechanical ventilation in COVID-19 pneumonia, European Heart Journal - Case Reports, Volume 4, Issue FI1, October 2020, Pages 1–2, https://doi.org/10.1093/ehjcr/ytaa213
301. Polistina GE, Lanza M, Di Somma C, Annunziata A, Fiorentino G. (2021). A Rare Evolution to Pneumopericardium in Patient with COVID-19 Pneumonia Treated with High Flow Nasal Cannula. Medicina (Kaunas). 2021 Oct 18;57(10):1122. doi: 10.3390/medicina57101122. PMID: 34684159; PMCID: PMC8539615.
302. A. Singh, J. Bass, and David H. Lindner (2020). Rare Complication of Pneumomediastinum and Pneumopericardium in a Patient with COVID-19 Pneumonia. Hindawi. Case Reports in Pulmonology. Volume 2020, Article ID 8845256, https://doi.org/10.1155/2020/8845256
303. Zhu H, Lieber JJ. (2020). COVID-19 and Spontaneous Pneumopericardium: A Case Report. Journal of Scientific Innovation in Medicine. 2020; 3(3): 4. DOI: https://doi.org/10.29024/jsim.57
304. K. T. Kadakia, A. L. Beckman, J. S. Ross (2021). Leveraging Open Science to Accelerate Research. March 24, 2021. DOI: 10.1056/NEJMp2034518
305. Worldometers- https://www.worldometers.info/coronavirus/#countries
306. Editorial from The New England Journal of Medicine (2020). Dying in a Leadership Vacuum. N Engl J Med 2020; 383:1479-1480. DOI: 10.1056/NEJMe2029812

307. W. E. Parmet (2021). Roman Catholic Diocese of Brooklyn v. Cuomo — The Supreme Court and Pandemic Controls. N Engl J Med 2021; 384:199-201. DOI: 10.1056/NEJMp2034280
308. Dellinger RP, Levy MM, Rhodes A et al. (2013). Surviving Sepsis Campaign Guidelines Committee including the Pediatric Subgroup. Surviving sepsis campaign: international guidelines for management of severe sepsis and septic shock: 2012. Crit Care Med. 2013 Feb;41(2):580-637. doi: 10.1097/CCM.0b013e31827e83af. PMID: 23353941.
309. Noritomi DT, Ranzani OT, Monteiro MB et al. (2014). Implementation of a multifaceted sepsis education program in an emerging country setting: clinical outcomes and cost-effectiveness in a long-term follow-up study. Intensive Care Med. 2014; 40: 182-191
310. A. Vidal, L. Santos (2017). Comorbidities impact on the prognosis of severe acute community-acquired pneumonia. Porto Biomedical Journal, Vol. 2. Num. 6. November - December 2017, pages 247-346
311. Yu KT, Wyer PC (2008). Evidence-based emergency medicine/ critically appraised topic. Evidence behind the 4-hour rule for initiation of antibiotic therapy in community-acquired pneumonia. Ann Emerg Med. 2008; 51: 651-662
312. Rider AC, Frazee BW. (2018). Community-Acquired Pneumonia. Emerg Med Clin North Am. 2018 Nov;36(4):665-683. doi: 10.1016/j.emc.2018.07.001. Epub 2018 Sep 6. PMID: 30296998; PMCID: PMC7126690.
313. Mohammad , A.K., Nasir, M., Paul, S., Rahman, H., Abul, K. and Ahmed, F.U. (2020). Common Pathogens and Their Resistance to Antimicrobials in Community Acquired Pneumonia (CAP): A Single Center Study in Bangladesh. International Journal of Medical Science and Clinical Invention. 7, 12 (Dec. 2020), 5144–5153. DOI:https://doi.org/10.18535/ijmsci/v7i12.04.
314. Montes-Andujar L, Tinoco E, Baez-Pravia O, et al. (2021). Empiric antibiotics for community-acquired pneumonia in adult patients: a systematic review and a network meta-analysis. Thorax 2021;76:1020-1031.
315. Koeckerling D, Barker J, Mudalige NL, et al. (2020). Awake prone positioning in COVID-19. Thorax Published Online First: 16 June 2020. doi: 10.1136/thoraxjnl-2020-215133

316. Thompson AE et al. (2020). Prone positioning in awake, nonintubated patients with COVID-19 hypoxemic respiratory failure. JAMA Intern Med 2020 Jun 17; [e-pub] (https://doi.org/10.1001/jamainternmed.2020.3030).

317. Tan W, Xu DY, Xu MJ, Wang ZF, Dai B, Li LL, Zhao HW, Wang W, Kang J. (2021). The efficacy and tolerance of prone positioning in non-intubation patients with acute hypoxemic respiratory failure and ARDS: a meta-analysis. Ther Adv Respir Dis. 2021 Jan-Dec;15:17534666211009407. doi: 10.1177/17534666211009407. PMID: 33888007; PMCID: PMC8071979.

318. Vianello A, Arcaro G, Molena B, et al. (2020). High-flow nasal cannula oxygen therapy to treat patients with hypoxemic acute respiratory failure consequent to SARS-CoV-2 infection. Thorax. Published Online First: 23 July 2020. doi: 10.1136/thoraxjnl-2020-214993

319. P. J. Young (2021). Effect of Oxygen Therapy on Mortality in the ICU. N Engl J Med 2021; 384:1361-1363. DOI: 10.1056/NEJMe2101538

320. Zhang X, Wang Y (2021). Comparison of outcomes of high-flow nasal cannula and noninvasive positive-pressure ventilation in patients with hypoxemia and various APACHE II scores after extubation. Ther Adv Respir Dis. 2021 Jan-Dec;15:17534666211004235. doi: 10.1177/17534666211004235. PMID: 33781130; PMCID: PMC8013886.

321. O. L. Schjørring, T. L. Klitgaard, A. Perner et al. (2021). Lower or Higher Oxygenation Targets for Acute Hypoxemic Respiratory Failure. N Engl J Med 2021; 384:1301-1311. DOI: 10.1056/NEJMoa2032510

322. R. Reddy, J. Dovidio, M. Baram et al. (2021). Outcomes of extracorporeal membrane oxygenation in ARDS due to COVID-19: comparison of the first and the second wave. Chest, Critical Care, Volume 160, Issue 4, Supplement , A1065, OCTOBER 01, 2021.DOI:https://doi.org/10.1016/j.chest.2021.07.985

323. Karagiannidis C, Mostert C, Hentschker C, et al. (2020). Case characteristics, resource use, and outcomes of 10 021 patients with COVID-19 admitted to 920 German hospitals: an observational study. Lancet Respir Med 2020;8:853-862.

324. Gavelli F, Castello LM, Avanzi GC. (2021). Management of sepsis and septic shock in the emergency department. Intern Emerg Med.

2021 Sep;16(6):1649-1661. doi: 10.1007/s11739-021-02735-7. Epub 2021 Apr 22. PMID: 33890208; PMCID: PMC8354945.

325. Evans, L., Rhodes, A., Alhazzani et al. (2021). Surviving sepsis campaign: international guidelines for management of sepsis and septic shock 2021. Intensive care medicine, 47(11), 1181–1247. https://doi.org/10.1007/s00134-021-06506-y
326. Shebl E, Paul M. (2021). Parapneumonic Pleural Effusions And Empyema Thoracis. 2021 Aug 11. In: StatPearls [Internet]. Treasure Island (FL): StatPearls Publishing; 2021 Jan–. PMID: 30485002.
327. Ceccato, A., Russo, A., Barbeta, E. et al. (2021). Real-world corticosteroid use in severe pneumonia: a propensity-score-matched study. Crit Care 25, 432 (2021). https://doi.org/10.1186/s13054-021-03840-x
328. L. A. Pérez de Llanoa, R. Golpea, D. Pérez-Ortiz et al. (2021). Early initiation of corticosteroids might be harmful in patients hospitalized with COVID-19 pneumonia: A multicenter propensity score analysis. Archivos de Bronconeumología. November 2021. https://doi.org/10.1016/j.arbres.2021.10.001
329. Angulo FJ, Finelli L, Swerdlow DL. (2021). Estimation of US SARS-CoV-2 infections, symptomatic infections, hospitalizations, and deaths using seroprevalence surveys. JAMA Netw Open 2021;4(1): e2033706-e2033706.
330. Reese H, Iuliano AD, Patel NN, et al. (2021). Estimated incidence of coronavirus disease 2019 (COVID-19) illness and hospitalization — United States, February–September 2020. Clin Infect Dis 2021;72(12):e1010-e1017.
331. Cilloniz C, Torres A, Niederman M S. (2021). Management of pneumonia in critically ill patients. BMJ, 2021; 375 :e065871, doi:10.1136/bmj-2021-065871
332. Bonneau E, Neveu B, Kostantin E, Tsongalis GJ, De Guire V. (2019). How close are miRNAs from clinical practice? A perspective on the diagnostic and therapeutic market. EJIFCC,2019;30:114-27.pmid:31263388
333. Gonzalo-Calvo D, de, Benítez ID, Pinilla L, et al. (2021). Circulating microRNA profiles predict the severity of COVID-19 in hospitalized patients. Transl Res,2021;236:147-59. doi:10.1016/j.trsl.2021.05.004.
334. Kyriazopoulou E, Karageorgos A, Liaskou-Antoniou L, et al. (2021). BioFire® FilmArray® pneumonia panel for severe lower respiratory

tract infections: subgroup analysis of a randomized clinical trial. Infect Dis Ther2021;10:1437-49. doi:10.1007/s40121-021-00459-x pmid:34120316

335. Arikan AA, Zappitelli M, Goldstein SL, Naipaul A, Jefferson LS, Loftis LL. (2012). Fluid overload is associated with impaired oxygenation and morbidity in critically ill children. Pediatr Crit Care Med. 2012;13(3):253–258pmid:21760565

336. Angus DC, Linde-Zwirble WT, Lidicker J, Clermont G, Carcillo J, Pinsky MR. (2001). Epidemiology of severe sepsis in the United States: analysis of incidence, outcome, and associated costs of care. Crit Care Med. 2001;29:1303–1310. doi: 10.1097/00003246-200107000-00002.

337. Kaukonen KM, Bailey M, Pilcher D, Cooper DJ, Bellomo R. (2015). Systemic inflammatory response syndrome criteria in defining severe sepsis. N Engl J Med. 2015;372:1629–1638. doi: 10.1056/NEJMoa1415236.

338. Montull B, Menendez R, Torres A, Reyes S, Mendez R, Zalacain R, et al.(2016). Predictors of severe sepsis among patients hospitalized for community-acquired pneumonia. PLoS One. 2016;11:e0145929. doi: 10.1371/journal.pone.0145929.

339. M. Ferrer, C. Travierso, C. Cilloniz et al. (2016). Severe community-acquired pneumonia: Characteristics and prognostic factors in ventilated and non-ventilated patients. Eur Respir J 2016; 48: Suppl. 60, 3025

340. Cao H, Han M, Li X, Dong S, Shang Y, Wang Q, Xu S and Liu j (2010), 'Clinical research evidence of cupping therapy in china: a systemic literature review', BMC complementary and Alternative Medicine, 10(70). [Online] Available at: http://www.biomedcentral.com/1472-6882/10/70(Accessed: 11 Jan 2013) DOI:10.1186/1472-6882-10-70

341. Farhadi K, Schwebelb D C, Saebc M, Choubsaza M, Mohammadid R and Ahmadi A (2009), 'The effectiveness of wet-cupping for nonspecific low back pain in Iran: A randomised controlled trial', Complementary Therapies in Medicine, 17(1), pp. 9-15. [Online] Available at: www.cebp.nl/vault_public/filesystem/?ID=3704 (Accessed: 25 Nov 2012) DOI:10.1016/j.ctim.2008.05.003

342. Kim, J.I. Lee, M.S. Lee, D.H. Boddy, K. and Ernst, E (2011) 'Cupping for treating pain: A systemic Review', Evidence-Based Complementary and Alternative Medicine, 2011. [Online] Available at:

http://www.hindawi.com/journals/ecam/2011/467014/ (Accessed: 16 Feb 2013) DOI: 10.1093/ecam/nep035

343. Lauche R, Cramer H, Hohmann C, Choi K E, Rampp T, Saha F J, Musial F, Langhorst J and Dobos G (2012), 'The effect of traditional cupping on pain and mechanical thresholds in patients with chronic Nonspecific neck pain: A randomised controlled pilot study', Evidence-Based Complementary and Alternative Medicine, 2012(2012). [Online]. Available at: http://www.hindawi.com/journals/ecam/2012/429718/ (Accessed: 25 Feb 2013) DOI: 10.1155/2012/429718

344. Vaskilampi T., Hanninen O. (1982), Cupping as an indigenous treatment of pain syndromes in Finnish culture and social context. Social science and Medicine, 16(21), pp. 1893-1901. [Online] Available at: http://www.sciencedirect.com/science/article/pii/0277953682904506 (Accessed: 24 Feb 2013) DOI: 10.1016/0277-9536(82)90450-6

345. Ahmadi, A. Schwebel, D.C. and Rezaei, M (2008) 'The Efficacy of wet-cupping in the treatment of tension and migraine headache', The American Journal of Chinese Medicine, 36(1), pp.37-44 [Online] Available at: http://tim.sums.ac.ir/icarusplus/export/sites/tim/journal-club/download/theefficacyofwecuppinginthetreatmentoftensionandmigraneheadache.pdf (Accessed: 02 Feb 2013)

346. Niasari, M. Kosari, F. and Ahmadi, A (2007) 'The effect of wet cupping on serum Lipid concentration of clinically healthy young men: A randomized controlled trial', The journal of Alternative and Complementary Medicine, 13(1), pp. 79-82. [Online] Available at: http://tim.sums.ac.ir/icarusplus/export/sites/tim/journal-club/download/theeffectofwetcuppingonserumlllipid.pdf (Accessed: 16 Feb 2013) DOI: 10.1089/acm.2006.4226

347. Ahmed, S.M. Madbouly, N.H. Maklad, S.S. and Abu-Shady, E.A (2005) 'Immunomodulatory effects of bloodletting cupping therapy in patients with Rheumatoid Arthritis', The Egyptian Journal of Immunology, 12(2), pp.39-51. [Online] Available at: http://www.dr-naseri.com/index.php?option=com_phocadownload&view=category&download=21:immunomodulatory-effects-of-blood-letting-cupping-therapy-in-patients-with-rheumatoid-arthritis&id=2& Itemid=75 (Accessed: 16 Feb 2013)

348. U.S. FDA (2016). Whole Body Cryotherapy (WBC): A "Cool" Trend that Lacks Evidence, Poses Risks. https://www.fda.gov/consumers/consumer-updates/whole-body-cryotherapy-wbc-cool-trend-lacks-evidence-poses-risks
349. Seetha Shankaran, Abbot R. Laptook, Richard A. Ehrenkranz et al. (2005). Whole-Body Hypothermia for Neonates with Hypoxic–Ischemic Encephalopathy. n engl j med 353;15. www.nejm.org ,october 13, 2005
350. Ur-Rahman S. (2012). Whole Body Hypothermia, Using Low Cost technique, is Safe and Effective in Term and Near-Term babies with Moderate and Severe Hypoxic Ischemic Encephalopathy. Journal of Clinical Neonatology. 2012 Jan;1(1):15-17. DOI: 10.4103/2249-4847.92236. PMID: 24027677; PMCID: PMC3761986.
351. Committee on fetus and newborn (2014). Hypothermia and Neonatal Encephalopathy. Pediatrics, June 2014, 133 (6) 1146-1150; DOI: https://doi.org/10.1542/peds.2014-0899
352. Ball MK, Hillman NH, Kallapur SG, et al. (2010). Body temperature effects on lung injury in ventilated preterm lambs. Resuscitation 2010; 81: 749–754.
353. Han HS, Park J, Kim JH, et al. (2012). Molecular and cellular pathways as a target of therapeutic hypothermia: pharmacological aspect. Curr Neuropharmacol 2012; 10: 80–87.
354. Pietrini D, Piastra M, Luca E, et al. (2012). Neuroprotection and hypothermia in infants and children. Curr Drug Targets 2012; 13: 925–935.
355. Suri LN, McCaig L, Picardi MV, et al. (2012). Adaptation to low body temperature influences pulmonary surfactant composition thereby increasing fluidity while maintaining appropriately ordered membrane structure and surface activity. Biochim Biophys Acta 2012; 1818: 1581–1589.
356. D. De Luca, S. Vázquez-Sánchez, A. Minucci et al. (2014). Effect of whole body hypothermia on inflammation and surfactant function in asphyxiated neonates. European Respiratory Journal Dec 2014, 44 (6) 1708-1710; DOI: 10.1183/09031936.00117714
357. Duan M, Berra L, Kumar A, et al. (2011). Use of hypothermia to allow low-tidal-volume ventilation in a patient with ARDS. Respir Care 2011; 56: 1956–1958.
358. Pietrini D, Pennisi M, Vitale F, et al. (2012). Rescue hypothermia for refractory hypercapnia. Eur J Pediatr 2012; 171: 1855–1857.

359. Igor Klepikov (2017). "Cupping therapy in the 21st century? - Why not!?".-Journal of General and Emergency Medicine, Vol 2,Issue 5
360. Igor Klepikov. "First Aid for Aggressive Forms of Acute Pneumonia". EC Pulmonology and Respiratory Medicine 7.2 (2018): 34-37.
361. Winearls S, Swingwood EL, Hardaker CL, et al. (2020). Early conscious prone positioning in patients with COVID-19 receiving continuous positive airway pressure: a retrospective analysis. BMJ, Open Respiratory Research, 2020;7:e000711. doi: 10.1136/bmjresp-2020-000711
362. Cordier J (2000). Organising pneumonia. Thorax 2000;55:318-328.
363. Schlesinger C, Koss MN. (2005). The organizing pneumonias: an update and review. Curr Opin Pulm Med. 2005 Sep;11(5):422-30. doi: 10.1097/01.mcp.0000175521.41729.07. PMID: 16093817.
364. M. B. Beasley (2010). The Pathologist's Approach to Acute Lung Injury. Arch Pathol Lab Med. 2010; 134:719–727
365. Cortés Colorado, J. M., Cardona Ardila, L. F., Aguirre Vásquez, N., Gómez Calderón, K. C., Lozano Álvarez, S. L., & Carrillo Bayona, J. A. (2021). Organizing pneumonia associated with SARS-CoV-2 infection. Radiology case reports, 16(9), 2634–2639. https://doi.org/10.1016/j.radcr.2021.06.028
366. Bieksiene, K., Zaveckiene, J., Malakauskas, K., Vaguliene, N., Zemaitis, M., & Miliauskas, S. (2021). Post COVID-19 Organizing Pneumonia: The Right Time to Interfere. Medicina (Kaunas, Lithuania), 57(3), 283. https://doi.org/10.3390/medicina57030283
367. Berkowitz's Pediatrics: A Primary Care Approach, 5th Edition Copyright © 2014 American Academy of Pediatrics p.537
368. Cough. https://en.wikipedia.org/wiki/Cough
369. Tuna, D. L., Ünal, M. A., Arı, F., Krumpe, P., and Evrensel, C. A. (June 1, 2020). "Enhancing Mucus Clearance by Cough Through Repeated Pulses." ASME. ASME J of Medical Diagnostics. August 2020; 3(3): 031004. https://doi.org/10.1115/1.4047188
370. Piva S, DiBlasi RM, Slee AE et al. (2021). Surfactant therapy for COVID-19 related ARDS: a retrospective case-control pilot study. Respir Res. 2021 Jan 18;22(1):20. doi: 10.1186/s12931-020-01603-w. PMID: 33461535; PMCID: PMC7812332.
371. A. V Bhansali and A. S. Shah (2021). "Physics of the Lung: Assessing the Role of Pulmonary Surfactants in COVID-19". EC Pulmonology and Respiratory Medicine 10.7 (2021): 08-12.

372. Veldhuizen RAW, Zuo YY, Petersen NO, Lewis JF, Possmayer F. (2021). The COVID-19 pandemic: a target for surfactant therapy? Expert Rev Respir Med. 2021 May;15(5):597-608. doi: 10.1080/17476348.2021.1865809. Epub 2020 Dec 28. PMID: 33331197.
373. Singh M, Singhi S, Walia BN. (1990). Evaluation of steam therapy in acute lower respiratory tract infections: a pilot study. Indian Pediatr. 1990 Sep;27(9):945-51. PMID: 2286438.
374. Little P, Moore M, Kelly J, Williamson I, Leydon G, McDermott L et al. (2013). Ibuprofen, paracetamol, and steam for patients with respiratory tract infections in primary care: pragmatic randomised factorial trial BMJ 2013; 347 :f6041 doi:10.1136/bmj.f6041
375. Baartmans, M., Kerkhof, E., Vloemans, J., Dokter, J., Nijman, S., Tibboel, D., & Nieuwenhuis, M. (2012). Steam inhalation therapy: severe scalds as an adverse side effect. The British journal of general practice : the journal of the Royal College of General Practitioners, 62(600), e473–e477. https://doi.org/10.3399/bjgp12X652337
376. NIH (2021). https://clinicaltrials.gov/ct2/show/NCT04743349
377. Klepikov I. Steamy inhalator. Patent No 1790416, USSR, 22.09.1992.
378. Klepikov I. Steamy inhalator. Bulletin of inventions, 1993; 3:77.
379. Klepikov I., Levina I., Mandrova R., Kazantseva V. The influence of steamy inhalator (Russian bath-house) on the cardiovascular system. At: The problems of professional pathology and individual health (reports of All Union Conference). Novokuznetsk, 1991; 85-87.
380. Levina I., Klepikov I., Mandrova R. Clinical and functional characteristic of patients with different forms of non-specific disease of lungs. At: Collection of scientific practical works by Kemerovo Regional Clinical Hospital, Kemerovo , 1993; 162-163.
381. http:// bigmed. info/ index. php/ microtracheostomy
382. Torrego, V. Pajares, C. Fernández-Arias et al. (2020). Bronchoscopy in Patients with COVID-19 with Invasive Mechanical Ventilation: A Single-Center Experience. American Journal of Respiratory and Critical Care Medicine, 202(2), pp. 284–287
383. Bruyneel M, Gabrovska M, Rummens P et al. (2020). Bronchoscopy in COVID-19 intensive care unit patients. Respirology. 2020 Dec;25(12):1313-1315. doi: 10.1111/resp.13932. Epub 2020 Aug 25. PMID: 32844524; PMCID: PMC7460941.

384. Widysanto A, Sutanto YS, Soetjipto AS, Lugito NP, Siahaan SS. (2020). Bronchoscopy Manifestation In Severe COVID-19 Patient: Case Series. Research Square; 2020. DOI: 10.21203/rs.3.rs-103263/v1.
385. Arenas-De Larriva, M., Martín-DeLeon, R., Urrutia Royo, B et al. (2021). The role of bronchoscopy in patients with SARS-CoV-2 pneumonia. ERJ open research, 7(3), 00165-2021. https://doi.org/10.1183/23120541.00165-2021
386. Manali E, Papadopoulos A, Tsiodras S, Polychronopoulos V, Giamarellou H, Kanellakopoulou K. (2008). The impact on community acquired pneumonia empirical therapy of diagnostic bronchoscopic techniques. Scand J Infect Dis. 2008;40(4):286-92. doi: 10.1080/00365540701663373. PMID: 17918018.
387. J. F. C. Duarte, C. R. Cordeiro, A. J. Ferreira (2016). Role of flexible-bronchoscopy in community-acquired pneumonia – A retrospective analysis. European Respiratory Journal, Sep 2016, 48 (suppl 60) PA2584; DOI: 10.1183/13993003.congress-2016.PA2584
388. Ranzani, O.T., Senussi, T., Idone, F. et al. (2019). Invasive and non-invasive diagnostic approaches for microbiological diagnosis of hospital-acquired pneumonia. Crit Care 23, 51 (2019). https://doi.org/10.1186/s13054-019-2348-2
389. C. O. Pickens, C. A. Gao, M. J. Cuttica etr al. (2021). Bacterial Superinfection Pneumonia in Patients Mechanically Ventilated for COVID-19 Pneumonia. American Journal of Respiratory and Critical Care Medicine, 204(8). DOI: 10.1164/rccm.202106-1354OC
390. Fengyun Wang, Bin Fang, LiXin Zhou et al. (2021). Severe 2019 novel coronavirus pneumonia may cause lung bullae and bronchiectasis: A case report and concise literature review. European Journal of Inflammation. Volume 19, 2021. https://doi.org/10.1177/20587392211029081
391. O'Brien KL, Baggett HC, Brooks WA, et al. (2019). Causes of severe pneumonia requiring hospital admission in children without HIV infection from Africa and Asia: the PERCH multi-country case-control study. Lancet. 2019; 394: 757- 779.
392. Weese W. C., Shindler E. R., Smith I. M., Rabinovich S. (1973). Empyema of the thorax then and now. A study of 122 cases over four decades. Arch Intern Med. 1973; 131: 516-520
393. Grijalva CG, Zhu Y, Nuorti JP, Griffin MR. (2011). Emergence of parapneumonic empyema in the USA. Thorax. 2011 Aug;66(8):663-

8. doi: 10.1136/thx.2010.156406. Epub 2011 May 26. PMID: 21617169; PMCID: PMC4820002.

394. Rosenstengel A. (2012). Pleural infection-current diagnosis and management. Journal of thoracic disease, 4(2), 186–193. https://doi.org/10.3978/j.issn.2072-1439.2012.01.12

395. Prasad R, Verma SK. (2005). A study of anaerobic infection in patients with empyema thoracis. J Int Med India 2005;8:75–9. (3

396. Maskell NA, Batt S, Hedley EL, et al. (2006). The bacteriology of pleural infection by genetic and standard methods and its mortality significance. Am J Respir Crit Care Med 2006;174:817–23.

397. C.F.N. Koegelenberg, A. H. Diacon. C. T. Bolliger (2008). Parapneumonic Pleural Effusion and Empyema. Respiration 2008;75:241–250 DOI: 10.1159/000117172

398. Sundaralingam, A., Banka, R. & Rahman, N.M. (2021). Management of Pleural Infection. Pulm Ther 7, 59–74 (2021). https://doi.org/10.1007/s41030-020-00140-7

399. Meyer, C.N., Armbruster, K., Kemp, M. et al. (2018). Pleural infection: a retrospective study of clinical outcome and the correlation to known etiology, co-morbidity and treatment factors. BMC Pulm Med 18, 160 (2018). https://doi.org/10.1186/s12890-018-0726-1

400. F. Jehan, I. Nisar, S. Kerai et al. (2020). Randomized Trial of Amoxicillin for Pneumonia in Pakistan. July 2, 2020. N Engl J Med 2020; 383:24-34 DOI: 10.1056/NEJMoa1911998

401. M Falguera, A Ruiz-Gonza´lez, J A Schoenenberger et al. (2010). Prospective, randomised study to compare empirical treatment versus targeted treatment on the basis of the urine antigen results in hospitalised patients with community-acquired pneumonia. . Thorax 2010 65: 101-106 originally published online August 23, 2009 doi: 10.1136/thx.2009.118588

402. Ferrer R, Martin-Loeches I, Phillips G, et al. (2014). Empiric antibiotic treatment reduces mortality in severe sepsis and septic shock from the first hour: results from a guideline-based performance improvement program. Crit Care Med. 2014;42(8):1749–1755pmid:24717459

403. Musher DM, Abers MS, Bartlett JG (2017). Evolving Understanding of the Causes of Pneumonia in Adults, With Special Attention to the Role of Pneumococcus. Clin Infect Dis. 2017;65(10):1736.

404. S. Jain, D. J. Williams, S. R. Arnold et al. (2015). Community-Acquired Pneumonia Requiring Hospitalization among U.S. Children. N Engl J Med 2015; 372:835-845 DOI: 10.1056/NEJMoa1405870
405. New CDC study highlights burden of pneumonia hospitalizations on U.S. children. Press Release.February 25, 2015. https://www.cdc.gov/media/releases/2015/p0225-pneumonia-hospitalizations.html
406. Gebistorf F, Karam O, Wetterslev J, Afshari A (2016) Inhaled nitric oxide for acute respiratory distress syndrome (ARDS) in children and adults. Cochrane Database Syst Rev 6:CD002787
407. Alhazzani, W., Møller, M.H., Arabi, Y.M. et al. (2020). Surviving Sepsis Campaign: guidelines on the management of critically ill adults with Coronavirus Disease 2019 (COVID-19). Intensive Care Med 46, 854–887 (2020). https://doi.org/10.1007/s00134-020-06022-5
408. Nonsteroidal anti-inflammatory drug. https://en.wikipedia.org/wiki/Nonsteroidal_anti-inflammatory_drug
409. Iizuka Y, Sanui M, Sasabuchi Y, et al. (2017). Low-dose immunoglobulin G is not associated with mortality in patients with sepsis and septic shock. Crit Care,2017;21:181. doi:10.1186/s13054-017-1764-4. pmid:28701223
410. Welte T, Dellinger RP, Ebelt H, et al. (2018). Efficacy and safety of trimodulin, a novel polyclonal antibody preparation, in patients with severe community-acquired pneumonia: a randomized, placebo-controlled, double-blind, multicenter, phase II trial (CIGMA study). Intensive Care Med,2018;44:438-48. doi:10.1007/s00134-018-5143-7 pmid:29632995
411. C. Salama, J. Han, L. Yau et al. (2020). Tocilizumab in Patients Hospitalized with Covid-19 Pneumonia. December 17, 2020. DOI: 10.1056/NEJMoa2030340
412. Roberta L. De Biasi (2021). Immunotherapy for MIS-C — IVIG, Glucocorticoids, and Biologics. N Engl J Med 2021; 385:74-75. DOI: 10.1056/NEJMe2108276
413. Keeling AN, Leong S, Logan PM, Lee MJ (2008). Empyema and effusion: outcome of imageguided small-bore catheter drainage. Cardiovasc Intervent Radiol 2008;31:135–141.
414. Cafarotti S., Dall'Armi V., Cusumano G. et al. (2011). Small-bore wire-guided chest drains: safety, tolerability, and effectiveness in

pneumothorax, malignant effusions, and pleural empyema. J Thorac Cardiovasc Surg. 2011; 141: 683-687

415. Havelock T, Teoh R, Laws D, et al. (2010). Pleural procedures and thoracic ultrasound: British Thoracic Society pleural disease guideline 2010 Thorax 2010;65:i61-i76.

416. F.J.H. Brims, S.M. Lansley, G.W. Waterer, Y.C.G. Lee (2010). Empyema thoracis: new insights into an old disease. European Respiratory Review 2010 19: 220-228; DOI: 10.1183/09059180.00005610

417. Islam S, Calkins CM, Goldin AB, Chen C, Downard CD, Huang EY, Cassidy L, Saito J, Blakely ML, Rangel SJ, Arca MJ, Abdullah F, St Peter SD; APSA Outcomes and Clinical Trials Committee, 2011-2012. The diagnosis and management of empyema in children: a comprehensive review from the APSA Outcomes and Clinical Trials Committee. J Pediatr Surg. 2012 Nov;47(11):2101-10. doi: 10.1016/j.jpedsurg.2012.07.047. PMID: 23164006.

418. Nehad AlFaraj., et al. (2022). "Necrotizing Pneumonia in an Infant, Case Report". EC Paediatrics 11.1 (2022): 10-18.

419. Harrington R. (2002) Necrotizing Pneumonia and Pulmonary Gangrene. In: Karmy-Jones R., Nathens A., Stern E.J. (eds) Thoracic Trauma and Critical Care. Springer, Boston, MA. https://doi.org/10.1007/978-1-4615-1127-4_53

420. Krishnadasan B, Sherbin VL, Vallières E, Karmy-Jones R. (2000). Surgical management of lung gangrene. Can Respir J. 2000 Sep-Oct;7(5):401-4. doi: 10.1155/2000/174703. PMID: 11058208.

421. Chatha, N., Fortin, D., & Bosma, K. J. (2014). Management of necrotizing pneumonia and pulmonary gangrene: a case series and review of the literature. Canadian respiratory journal, 21(4), 239–245. https://doi.org/10.1155/2014/864159

422. Refaely Y, Weissberg D. (1997). Gangrene of the lung: treatment in two stages. Ann Thorac Surg. 1997 Oct;64(4):970-3; discussion 973-4. doi: 10.1016/s0003-4975(97)00837-0. PMID: 9354511.

423. Reimel BA, Krishnadasen B, Cuschieri J, Klein MB, Gross J, Karmy-Jones R. (2006). Surgical management of acute necrotizing lung infections. Can Respir J. 2006; 13:369–73.

424. W. H.Chong, B.K.Saha, E.Conuel et al. (2021). The incidence of pleural effusion in COVID-19 pneumonia: State-of-the-art review. Heart & Lung, Volume 50, Issue 4, July–August 2021, Pages 481-490

425. Şatir Türk M, Akarsu I, Tombul I, et al. (2021). Pleural complications of Covid-19 pneumonia. Turkish Journal of Medical Sciences. 2021 Apr. DOI: 10.3906/sag-2012-268. PMID: 33890447.
426. Fox S.E., Akmatbekov A., Harbert J.L. et al. (2020). Pulmonary and cardiac pathology in African American patients with COVID-19: an autopsy series from New Orleans. Lancet Respir Med. 2020;8(7):681–686. doi: 10.1016/S2213-2600(20)30243-5.
427. Menter T, Haslbauer JD, Nienhold R et al. (2020). Postmortem examination of COVID-19 patients reveals diffuse alveolar damage with severe capillary congestion and variegated findings in lungs and other organs suggesting vascular dysfunction. Histopathology. 2020;77(2):198–209. https://doi.org/10.1111/his.14134.
428. Yao XH, Li TY, He ZC, Ping YF et al. (2020). A pathological report of three COVID-19 cases by minimal invasive autopsies. Zhonghua Bing Li Xue Za Zhi. 2020;49(5):411–7. https://doi.org/10.3760/cma.j.cn112151-20200312-00193.
429. Hidron, A., Quiceno, W., Cardeño, J. J., Roncancio, G., & García, C. (2021). Post-COVID-19 Necrotizing Pneumonia in Patients on Invasive Mechanical Ventilation. Infectious disease reports, 13(3), 835–842. https://doi.org/10.3390/idr13030075
430. Carsana L., Sonzogni A., Nasr A. et al. (2020). Pulmonary post-mortem findings in a series of COVID-19 cases from northern Italy: A two-centre descriptive study. Lancet Infect. Dis. 2020;20:1135–1140. doi: 10.1016/S1473-3099(20)30434-5.
431. Nicolaou EV, Bartlett AH. (2017). Necrotizing Pneumonia. Pediatr Ann. 2017 Feb 1;46(2):e65-e68. doi: 10.3928/19382359-20170120-02. PMID: 28192581.
432. Carpio-Orantes L D. (2017). Necrotizing pneumonia or pulmonary gangrene. Community Acquir Infect 2017;4:56-8
433. D. Sekarsari, S. Handoyo, M. YanuarAmal et al. (2021). Necrotizing pneumonia with bronchopleural fistula as an uncommon complication of pneumonia in children: a case report. Radiology Case Reports, Volume 16, Issue 8, August 2021, Pages 2077-2080
434. Peeters, K., Mesotten, D., Willaert, X., Deraedt, K., Nauwelaers, S., & Lauwers, G. (2021). Salvage Lobectomy to Treat Necrotizing SARS-CoV-2 Pneumonia Complicated by a Bronchopleural Fistula. The Annals of thoracic surgery, 111(4), e241–e243. https://doi.org/10.1016/j.athoracsur.2020.10.038

435. Nizami M, Grieco C, Hogan J, et al. (2021). Surgical management of a COVID-19-associated necrotic pneumonia. BMJ, Case Reports CP, 2021;14:e240766.
436. Oye M, Ali A, Kandah F, Chowdhury N. (2020). Two cases of spontaneous pneumomediastinum with pneumothorax in patients with COVID-19 associated pneumonia. Respiratory Medicine Case Reports 2020; 31: 101308. doi: 10.1016/j.rmcr.2020.101308
437. Song F., Shi N., Shan F. (2020). Emerging 2019 novel coronavirus (2019-nCoV) pneumonia. Radiology. 2020;295(1):210–217. doi: 10.1148/radiol.2020200274.
438. Han R., Huang L., Jiang H. et al. (2020). Early clinical and CT manifestations of coronavirus disease 2019 (COVID-19) Pneumonia. Published online 2020:6. [PubMed]
439. Wang Y., Dong C., Hu Y. (2020). Temporal changes of CT findings in 90 patients with COVID-19 pneumonia: a longitudinal study. Radiology. 2020;296(2):E55–E64. doi: 10.1148/radiol.2020200843.
440. Evidence-based medicine. https://en.wikipedia.org/wiki/Evidence-based_medicine
441. Evidence-Based Medicine Working Group (November 1992). "Evidence-based medicine. A new approach to teaching the practice of medicine". JAMA. 268 (17): 2420–25. Cite Seer X 10.1.1.684. 3783. doi:10.1001/JAMA.1992.03490170092032. PMID 1404801.
442. Sackett DL, Rosenberg WM, Gray JA, Haynes RB, Richardson WS (1996). "Evidence based medicine: what it is and what it isn't". BMJ. 312 (7023): 71–72. doi:10.1136/bmj.312.7023.71. PMC 2349778. PMID 8555924.
443. Cavallazzi R, Furmanek S, Arnold FW, et al. (2020). The burden of community-acquired pneumonia requiring admission to ICU in the United States. Chest,2020;158:1008-16.
doi:10.1016/j.chest.2020.03.051 pmid:32298730
444. Hoffmann, J., Machado, D., Terrier et al. (2016). Viral and bacterial co-infection in severe pneumonia triggers innate immune responses and specifically enhances IP-10: a translational study. Scientific reports, 6, 38532. https://doi.org/10.1038/srep38532
445. Kamat IS, Ramachandran V, Eswaran H, Guffey D, Musher DM. (2020). Procalcitonin to Distinguish Viral From Bacterial Pneumonia: A Systematic Review and Meta-analysis. Clin Infect Dis. 2020 Jan 16;70(3):538-542. doi: 10.1093/cid/ciz545. PMID: 31241140.

446. Marik PE, Iglesias J, Voron, Kory P. (2021). COVID-19 In-Hospital Mortality: A Concise Worldwide Review. J Comm Med And Pub Health Rep 2(4): Https://Doi.Org/10.38207/Jcmphr20210073
447. Wang D, Hu B, Hu C, et al. (2020). Clinical characteristics of 138 hospitalized patients with 2019 novel coronavirus-infected pneumonia in Wuhan, China. JAMA 2020;323:1061–doi:10.1001/jama.2020.1585pmid:http://www.ncbi.nlm.nih.gov/pubmed/32031570
448. Ponsford MJ, Jefferies R, Davies C, et al. (2021). Burden of nosocomial COVID-19 in Wales: results from a multicentre retrospective observational study of 2508 hospitalised adults. Thorax 2021. doi:doi:10.1136/thoraxjnl-2021-216964.
449. Huang C, Wang Y, Li X, Ren L, Zhao J, Hay, et al. (2020). Clinical features of patients infected with 2019 novel coronavirus in Wuhan, China. Lancet, 2020;395:497-506.
450. Yu Y, Xu D, Fu S, Zhang J, Yang X, Xu L, et al. (2020). Patients with COVID-19 in 19 ICUs in Wuhan, China: A cross-sectional study. Crit Care 2020; 24:219.
451. Berenguer J, Borobia AM, Ryan P, et al. (2021). Development and validation of a prediction model for 30-day mortality in hospitalised patients with COVID-19: the COVID-19 SEIMC score. Thorax Published Online First: 25 February 2021. doi: 10.1136/thoraxjnl-2020-216001
452. Chua F, Vancheeswaran R, Draper A, et al. ((2021). Early prognostication of COVID-19 to guide hospitalisationtion versus outpatient monitoring using a point-of-test risk prediction score. Thorax 2021; 76:696-703.
453. Ruetzler K, Szarpak Ł, Ładny JR, et al. (2021). D-dimer levels predict COVID-19 severity and mortality. Kardiolardiol Pol. 2021; 79: 217-218. doi:10.33963/KP.15830
454. Knight SR, Gupta RK, Ho A, et al. (2021). Prospective validation of the 4C prognostic models for adults hospitaospitalised with COVID-19 using the ISARIC WHO Clinical Characterisation Protocol. Thorax, Published Online First: 22 November 2021. doi: 10.1136/thoraxjnl-2021-217629
455. Angélica Jayk Bernal, Monica M. Gomes da Silva, Danny B. Musungaie et al., for the MOVe-OUT Study Group (2021). Molnupiravir for Oral Treatment of Covid-19 in Nonhospitalized Patients. December 16, 2021. DOI: 10.1056/NEJMoa2116044

456. M. Esperatti,M. Busico,N. Fuentes et al. (2022). Impact of exposure time in awake prone positioning on clinical outcomes of patients with COVID-19-related acute respiratory failure treated with high-flow nasal oxygen: a multicenter cohort study. Open Access. Critical Care, (2022) 26:16 https://doi.org/10.1186/s13054-021-03881-2

457. Rudd KE, Johnson SC, Agesa KM et al. (2020). Global, regional, and national sepsis incidence and mortality, 1990–2017: analysis for the Global Burden of Disease Study. Lancet 395(10219):200–211

458. Wang H.E., Jones A.R., Donnelly J.P. (2017). Revised national estimates of emergency department visits for sepsis in the United States. Crit Care Med. 2017; 45: 1443-1449

459. CDC. Сепсис. Clinical Information. Surveillance and Epidemiology. August 2018. https://www.cdc.gov/sepsis/clinicaltools/index.html?CDC_AA_refVal=https%3A%2F%2Fwww.cdc.gov%2Fsepsis%2Fdatareports%2Findex.html

460. Rhee C.,Jones T.M.,Hamad Y.et al.(2019). Prevalence, underlying causes, and preventability of sepsis-associated mortality in US acute care hospitals. JAMA, Netw Open. 2019; 2e187571

461. Fleischmann C, ScheragA, Adhikari NK, et al. (2016). Assessment of global incidence and mortality of hospital-treated sepsis. Current estimates and limitations. Am J Respir Crit Care Med. 2016;193(3): 259–272. doi: 10.1164/rccm.201504-0781OC.

462. Rhee C, Dantes R, Epstein L, et al. (2017). Incidence and trends of sepsis in US hospitals using clinical vs claims data, 2009–2014. JAMA. 2017;318(13):1241–1249. doi: 10.1001/jama.2017.13836.

463. Fleischmann-Struzek C, Mellhammar L, RoseN, et al. (2020). Incidence and mortality of hospital- and ICU-treated sepsis: results from an updated and expanded systematic review and meta-analysis. Intensive Care Med. 2020;46(8):1552–1562. doi: 10.1007/s00134-020-06151-x.

464. Angus DC, Barnato AE, Bell D, et al. (2015). A systematic review and meta-analysis of early goal-directed therapy for septic shock: the ARIS, ProCESS and ProMISe Investigators. Intensive Care Med, 2015;41:1549-60.

465. File TM Jr, Marrie TJ. (2010). Burden of community-acquired pneumonia in North American adults. Postgrad Med. 2010 Mar;122(2):130-41.
doi: 10.3810/pgm.2010.03.2130. PMID: 20203464.

466. Broulette J, Yu H, Pyenson B, Iwasaki K, Sato R. (2013). The incidence rate and economic burden of community-acquired pneumonia in a working-age population. Am Health Drug Benefits. 2013, Sep;6(8):494-503. PMID: 24991378; PMCID: PMC4031734.
467. Centers for Disease Control and Prevention. National Center for Health Statistics. Pneumonia. http://www.cdc.gov/nchs/fastats/pneumonia.htm. Accessed January 18, 2016.
468. Kaysin A, Viera AJ. (2016). Community-Acquired Pneumonia in Adults: Diagnosis and Management. Am Fam Physician. 2016 Nov 1;94(9):698-706. Erratum in: Am Fam Physician. 2017 Apr 1;95(7):414. PMID: 27929242.
469. Meme. https://en.wikipedia.org/wiki/Meme
470. Easley D. (2010). Networks, Crowds and Markets: Reasoning about a Highly Connected World. Cambridge University Press. Chapter 16.
471. Heffron R. (1939). Pneumonia, with special reference to pneumococcus lobar pneumonia. Cambridge: Harvard University Press; 1939.
472. Small JT. (1948). A short history of the pneumococcus with special reference to lobar pneumonia. Edinb Med J. 1948;55(3):129–41.
473. Shoar, S., Musher, D.M. (2020). Etiology of community-acquired pneumonia in adults: a systematic review. Pneumonia 12, 11 (2020). https://doi.org/10.1186/s41479-020-00074-3
474. Cilloniz, C., Martin-Loeches, I., Garcia-Vidal, C., San Jose, A., & Torres, A. (2016). Microbial Etiology of Pneumonia: Epidemiology, Diagnosis and Resistance Patterns. International journal of molecular sciences, 17(12), 2120. https://doi.org/10.3390/ijms17122120
475. Jeremiah SS, Miyakawa K, Morita T, Yamaoka Y, Ryo A. (2020). Potent antiviral effect of silver nanoparticles on SARS-CoV-2. Biochem Biophys Res Commun. 2020 Nov 26;533(1):195-200. doi: 10.1016/j.bbrc.2020.09.018. Epub 2020 Sep 11. PMID: 32958250; PMCID: PMC7486059.
476. Reznikov, L. R., Norris, M. H., Vashisht, R., Bluhm, A. P., Li, D., Liao, Y. J., Brown, A., Butte, A. J., & Ostrov, D. A. (2021). Identification of antiviral antihistamines for COVID-19 repurposing. Biochemical and biophysical research communications, 538, 173–179. https://doi.org/10.1016/j.bbrc.2020.11.095

477. Budak GG, Özkan S, Budak M, Sekret, Meryemoglu B, Miron SS, et al. (2022). Preclinical toxicity test results of a new antiviral–immune-modulator compound consisting of flavonoid molecules (COVID-19 clinical trial preliminary data). Explore Med. 2022;3:1–21. https://doi.org/10.37349/emed.2022.00071

478. R. J. Baron, Y. D. Eines (2022). Physicians Spreading Misinformation on Social Media — Do Right and Wrong Answers Still Exist in Medicine? NEJM, May 18, 2022. DOI: 10.1056/NEJMp2204813